Praise for *The Teacher's Guide to Restorative Yoga*

"*The Teacher's Guide to Restorative Yoga* is not only a visually beautiful book, it is also a persuasive and important contribution to the field of Restorative Yoga. With figures and clear text, Audrey Favreau shows us both the inner and outer beauty of the practice of deep and conscious resting. There could not be a better time to incorporate the poses this book offers into your yoga practice and life."

—JUDITH HANSON LASATER, PhD, PT, yoga teacher since 1971 and author of ten books, including *Yoga Myths*

"In a world increasingly governed by the doṣa Vāta, everyone longs for peace of mind and a grounded connection to the earth. 'Stop and observe,' taught Zen master Thich Nhat Hanh. Audrey Favreau's book, *The Teacher's Guide to Restorative Yoga*, offers us a powerful invitation to embody mindfulness through stillness and presence. Her book is an offering of compassion in action—rich in insight and rooted in lived experience."

—FRANÇOIS RAOULT, MA, E-RYT500, C-IAYT, author of *My Lifāsana*

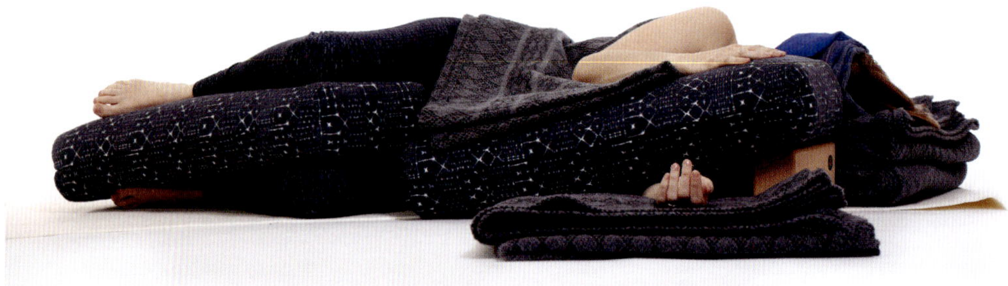

Side-Lying Savasana with full-body support: Head, upper body, knees, and ankles are cushioned for deep rest.

THE TEACHER'S GUIDE TO Restorative Yoga

30+ THERAPEUTIC POSE AND SEQUENCE COMBINATIONS
to Calm *the* Nervous System, Access Deep Rest, *and* Achieve Hormonal Balance

---

AUDREY FAVREAU

FOREWORD BY LIZZIE LASATER

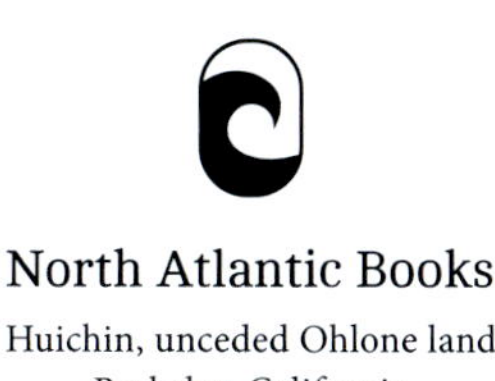

North Atlantic Books
Huichin, unceded Ohlone land
Berkeley, California

North Atlantic Books
Huichin, unceded Ohlone land
2526 Martin Luther King Jr Way
Berkeley, CA 94704 USA
www.northatlanticbooks.com

Cover art © Jill via Adobe Stock
Cover design by Jasmine Hromjak
Book design by Happenstance Type-O-Rama
Photos by Carlo Cattadori

Printed in the United States of America

The Teacher's Guide to Restorative Yoga: 30+ Therapeutic Pose and Sequence Combinations to Calm the Nervous System, Access Deep Rest, and Achieve Hormonal Balance is sponsored and published by North Atlantic Books, an educational nonprofit that collaborates with partners to develop cross-cultural perspectives; nurture holistic views of art, science, the humanities, and healing; and seed personal and global transformation by publishing work on the relationship of body, spirit, and nature.

North Atlantic Books's publications are distributed to the US trade and internationally by Penguin Random House Publisher Services. For further information, visit our website at www.northatlanticbooks.com.

The authorized representative in the EU for product safety and compliance is Eucomply OÜ, Pärnu mnt 139b-14, 11317 Tallinn, Estonia, hello@eucompliancepartner.com, +33757690241.

MEDICAL DISCLAIMER: The following information is intended for general information purposes only. Individuals should always see their health care provider before administering any suggestions made in this book. Any application of the material set forth in the following pages is at the reader's discretion and is their sole responsibility.

Library of Congress Cataloging-in-Publication Data

Names: Favreau, Audrey author
Title: The teacher's guide to restorative yoga : 30+ therapeutic pose and sequence combinations to calm the nervous system, access deep rest, and achieve hormonal balance / Audrey Favreau ; Foreword by Lizzie Lasater.
Description: Berkeley, California : North Atlantic Books, [2026] | Includes bibliographical references. | Summary: "A complete guide to restorative yoga that includes 40 adaptable yoga sequences"— Provided by publisher.
Identifiers: LCCN 2026000567 (print) | LCCN 2026000568 (ebook) | ISBN 9798889843702 trade paperback | ISBN 9798889843719 ebook
Subjects: LCSH: Hatha yoga—Study and teaching
Classification: LCC RA781.67 .F38 2026 (print) | LCC RA781.67 (ebook)
LC record available at https://lccn.loc.gov/2026000567
LC ebook record available at https://lccn.loc.gov/2026000568

1 2 3 4 5 6 7 8 9 VERSA 30 29 28 27 26

To Giorgio Léon and Alessandro Carlo,

Who you are matters more than what you do. May you always make space to simply be—to rest, to feel, to breathe. Care for your body with tenderness. It carries your soul.

With all my love,

Maman

Contents

Foreword

I used to think Restorative Yoga was boring.

As a kid in the 1990s, I spent summer afternoons wandering around yoga retreat centers while my mother, Restorative Yoga pioneer Judith Hanson Lasater, taught. During the afternoon sessions, I remember watching the clock, horrified that adults would choose to lie around over bolsters for hours.

How boring!

Now I understand: This practice isn't boring. It's brave. Restorative Yoga invites us into a radically different relationship with time. It gently challenges the myth that we must always be productive. In stillness, we don't shut down. We open up: to intuition, to creativity, to a deeper kind of listening.

As a working mother and yoga content creator, I rely on Restorative Yoga not just to recover, but to generate. Rest becomes the ground of my ideas, my teaching, my connection to others. The poses create a kind of internal spaciousness; a blank space from which something new can arise.

My mom writes in *Restore and Rebalance* that Restorative Yoga is "quieting and pacifying to a ragged nervous system and weary mind."[1] She's right. But I'd add that this practice is also profoundly creative. It's not about napping; it's about allowing your system to downshift so that your inner insight arises.

We have many methods to soothe ourselves: a glass of wine, a hot bath, the endless scroll through our phones. But Restorative Yoga is different. It's conscious. Nourishing. And it teaches us how to soften into presence, even when the world feels precarious.

In *The Teacher's Guide to Restorative Yoga*, Audrey Favreau offers an intelligent and practical guide to this essential form. Audrey is a dedicated and sincere practitioner whose teaching arises from years of personal practice and embodied study. Whether you are new to Restorative Yoga or returning to it with fresh eyes, I hope this book helps you experience that sweet, sacred pause where rest and creativity meet.

LIZZIE LASATER

Salzburg, 2025

Preface

I clearly remember my first yoga class. I was six years old and accompanying my mother to hers. I tried to follow the teacher's instructions, but experiencing the effects of a pose on one side of my body and then noticing the difference before switching sides left me confused. At the time, I decided yoga wasn't for me. Yet that moment stayed with me, like a seed quietly planted deep within.

As a child, I experienced emotional abuse and chronic stress, and as a young adult, I struggled with anxiety and panic attacks while navigating life in a French business school and later traveling the globe for a large bank. I tried nearly everything, except yoga, to manage my stress: relaxation techniques like sophrology, meditation, embodied practices like qigong, dance, reflexology, and psychotherapy, which I began in 2006. Despite my efforts, the concept of "letting go" remained elusive. My only strategy was to maintain control over every aspect of my life. That was how I had been taught—by my parents, at school, at work, and by society. There were no shortcuts to success; I had to work hard and control everything. By age thirty I was managing over forty people at a large French bank. Yet despite all my achievements, I couldn't fulfill my most cherished dream—becoming a mother.

I suffered from endometriosis, which caused intense menstrual pain. Medical treatments and adoption attempts failed. Physically I felt constant pressure in my chest, and my breath was irregular, as if I was perpetually holding it. Emotionally I was deeply depressed. Later I discovered that this state is described in the Yoga Sutras of Patanjali as symptoms of a life overwhelmed by afflictions: "Pain, despair, nervousness, and disordered inspiration and expiration are the symptoms of a distracted condition of mind."[1]

In 2011, I began a master's program in coaching, intending to support the growth of my employees. Instead it became a transformative journey of personal growth for me. This program not only provided me with the tools to navigate a painful divorce but, more profoundly, compelled me to confront the reality that my reliance on control had ultimately failed. It was through this realization that I finally grasped the true essence of letting go: Control was nothing more than an illusion.

Learning to let go was far from easy, especially as I was in the process of rebuilding my life. Old habits lingered, and the struggle to find balance between effort and overexertion often left me drained and defeated. But little by little, I chose to place my trust in the universe and embrace what it offered. In return, I was given an unexpected gift: a sense of ease, the first step toward breaking free from the patterns that had held me back for so long.

In 2012 I discovered Restorative Yoga during a trip to Bali. (It wasn't yet available in France.) It was love at first sight. In just a few minutes I could relax deeply and experience sensations so comforting that they felt revolutionary. This practice became my daily anchor, helping me let go physically, mentally, and emotionally. It was nothing short of transformative. Restorative Yoga has remained a steadfast companion in my life, offering the unwavering reassurance that the earth is always there to support me. Guided by this sense of grounding, I traveled alone, a journey that allowed me to reconnect with myself and uncover my truest desires. I met my future husband in Rome, left my banking job, moved to Italy, and devoted myself to developing and sharing Restorative Yoga across Europe and worldwide, thanks to my online platform. Along the way I became the mother of two lively boys.

Since 2014, I have studied continuously with renowned teachers, including Judith Hanson Lasater, Bo Forbes, François Raoult, Jillian Pransky, Donna Farhi, Robert Svoboda, and Edwin F. Bryant. Through their guidance and wisdom I have deepened my understanding of yoga and its transformative power. The daily practice of Restorative Yoga has profoundly shaped my life, teaching me to slow down, embrace stillness, and develop a heightened awareness of my patterns and emotions. This practice has become a cornerstone of my personal growth and well-being.

This practice has been profoundly transformative. It has taught me to soften the edges of reactivity, to pause and breathe before responding, and to meet life's intensity with greater clarity and calm. It has guided me toward a place of moderation—where I can create space between a stimulus and my response, and choose more consciously how I show up. Most importantly, it has helped me recognize, acknowledge, and honor my most vulnerable emotions and unmet needs without judgment. This is not a path toward perfection—there are still moments when I react in ways I later regret. But the difference now lies in how I relate to myself afterward: with self-empathy, tenderness, and the growing ability to stay present even in my imperfection.

I hope this book inspires you to explore this practice, whether on your own or with a qualified yoga teacher. Restorative Yoga is a beautiful practice, but it can feel inaccessible at first. Our bodies, minds, and emotions often carry so much tension that relaxation might seem impossible. In the beginning, your mind might race, fixating on physical discomfort, emotions, or worries. Do not let these initial experiences discourage you. Be patient and trust the process.

With consistent practice, by the third or fourth day, you'll notice your mind beginning to settle and your physical tensions starting to melt away. Though new challenges may emerge, they will be met with a growing sense of calm and balance, perhaps a feeling unlike anything you've experienced before. You'll become acutely aware of the tensions you've carried for years, recognizing them as gentle reminders that it is time to prioritize your well-being and truly take care of yourself.

I often compare Restorative Yoga to peeling the layers of an onion. With each practice, we gently shed the layers of tension, old wounds, and deep-seated emotions, gradually revealing our truest, most authentic selves. The more you nurture and care for yourself, the more energy, compassion, and empathy you'll have to offer others. Each practice becomes a gift, not only to yourself but also to those around you, as you show up fully present and aligned with your most genuine self.

Wishing you a deeply soothing and transformative practice!

Acknowledgments

This book is the culmination of a journey that would not have been possible without the invaluable guidance, support, and inspiration of many people.

To my teachers, Judith Hanson Lasater, François Raoult, and Bo Forbes: thank you for your profound wisdom and generosity. I am especially grateful to Judith Hanson Lasater and François Raoult for their unwavering support and encouragement throughout my journey. Restorative Yoga has become a cornerstone of my life and the lives of many of my students, who continue to share this practice with love and dedication.

Finally, and most importantly, to my husband, Guido Parodi: thank you for your unwavering love, patience, and the countless hours you devoted to caring for our children while I focused on bringing these pages to life. Your belief in me made this possible, and for that, I am forever grateful.

To all who have contributed to this journey, directly or indirectly, my heartfelt thanks.

CHAPTER 1

Where Does Restorative Yoga Come From?

The Pioneers: B. K. S. Iyengar and Judith Hanson Lasater

In the sixth chapter of the Bhagavad Gita, one of Hinduism's most important texts, the word *sapasraye* is used. According to Acharya Ramanuja, it means "hanging on, leaning against, depending upon, support." This concept of support finds a parallel in modern Restorative Yoga, pioneered by B. K. S. Iyengar, a globally respected authority on yoga who died in 2014.

B. K. S. Iyengar's Innovations

Iyengar's dedication to refining his yoga practice led him to innovate using makeshift props like sticks and bricks he found on the road. These simple tools enabled him to delve deeper into the exploration and perfection of asanas. Over time, he recognized that these "supporters" not only enhanced the learning process but also made it possible to master even the most complex poses with greater accessibility and precision.[1]

After establishing his institute in Pune, India, Iyengar noticed that while his guidance often brought students immediate relief, the benefits rarely lasted when they practiced on their own. Without external support, many found it difficult to sustain poses effectively, leading to the recurrence of their issues.

To address this, Iyengar systematically designed and adjusted props tailored to individual needs. Props enabled students to:

- perform challenging asanas with confidence and minimal strain.
- hold poses longer, reducing stress and muscle tension.
- build independence and practice free of pain.

These innovations included chairs, slanting planks, and bricks, while hanging ropes reflected a legacy from his guru. By enhancing circulation, improving respiratory function, and amplifying the therapeutic effects of yoga, props became integral to Iyengar's method.

In 1993, during a yoga teachers convention in the United States, Iyengar introduced a sequence of twelve restorative poses to help participants recover from an intense program. This marked the essence of modern Restorative Yoga: It is adaptable, effective, and deeply nourishing.

A Critical Look at the Legacy

While B. K. S. Iyengar's influence on modern yoga is undeniably significant, it is also important to acknowledge the more complex aspects of his teaching style. Over the years, several respected voices in the yoga community have brought attention to a culture of authoritarianism and even abuse that emerged around his methods.[2] Donna Farhi, an internationally respected yoga teacher and former student of Iyengar, has spoken publicly about her experience of being physically assaulted by him during a class. In her reflections, shared in interviews and public talks such as "Iyengar Abuse and Changing Yoga Pedagogy,"[3] she describes a broader teaching culture that normalized shouting, hitting, and pushing students beyond their limits. Such methods were often seen as necessary for transformation, but in many cases, they crossed the line into coercion and trauma. Farhi also draws attention to systemic issues that enabled these behaviors: the lack of clear boundaries, the assumption of implied consent, and the concentration of authority in the hands of the teacher. These dynamics can create environments where students feel powerless and unable to speak up or protect their own well-being.

Critique of the Iyengar lineage deepened with the case of Manouso Manos, a senior teacher accused of sexual misconduct since the 1980s, whose complaints were routinely mishandled, often by ethics committees involving his own students. Farhi highlighted the systemic resistance to accountability within the Iyengar organization, especially in India, where hierarchical structures and institutional nepotism silenced victims and deterred dissent. She also exposed a wider pattern of abuse, including violent physical adjustments that caused serious injuries, some of which she experienced personally. Recognizing these harmful patterns does not erase Iyengar's contributions. Rather, it encourages us to build on his legacy with greater ethical awareness. It also points to the vital role of Restorative Yoga as a healing response, not only to the fast pace of modern life but also to the harm that can sometimes arise within yoga itself.

Restorative Yoga offers a different path. Instead of effort, violence, and authority, it emphasizes safety, stillness, and deep listening. It places consent at the center of the practice, nurtures autonomy, and gently restores the practitioner's inner sense of trust and agency. For students who carry physical, sexual, or emotional scars, including those from previous yoga experiences, Restorative Yoga can become both a refuge and a path toward profound healing. It is no coincidence, then, that Judith Hanson Lasater, one of Iyengar's most dedicated students, chose to distance herself from the more forceful elements of his teaching. In developing Restorative Yoga, she shaped a practice rooted in gentleness, deep support, and nonintervention. Her approach honors the intelligence of the body and prioritizes the student's inner experience above all else.

Judith Hanson Lasater's Contributions

Judith Hanson Lasater played a pivotal role in introducing Restorative Yoga to the United States. Her seminal 1995 book, *Relax and Renew*, brought this gentle and nourishing practice to wider audience, laying the foundation for its steady and meaningful growth. Lasater's personal journey with Restorative Yoga deepened after the loss of her twin brother on their forty-fifth birthday. Finding solace in Supta Baddha Konasana (Reclining Bound Angle Pose, fig. 4.1), she spent an hour in the pose every day for a year. In that quiet space she described feeling "simultaneously open and supported, free and comforted, soft and expansive." It was this lived experience of rest as refuge that inspired her to share the healing potential of Restorative Yoga with others.

Building on Iyengar's use of props, Lasater refined the practice into a gentle, meditative form of yoga that invites the body into deep rest. Poses are typically held for extended periods, between five and thirty minutes, supported by bolsters, blankets, and other props to eliminate strain and encourage complete surrender. More than a physical technique, this receptive approach nurtures the whole being: body, mind, and heart. Rather than asking the body to do more, Restorative Yoga invites it to soften, to listen, and simply to be. In this stillness, healing unfolds, not through effort or striving but through the quiet power of presence, surrender, and deep inner listening.

The Purpose of Restorative Yoga

At its core, Restorative Yoga aims to calm the nervous system by shifting the body from sympathetic dominance (fight or flight) to parasympathetic dominance (rest and digest). This shift not only aids digestion but also helps process the sensory impressions we encounter daily: what we see, hear, and feel. Through this process, we assimilate what nourishes us and release the tensions that hinder our well-being.

The practice also opens the door to healing emotional pain. Sometimes this suffering manifests physically, such as tightness or constriction around the heart. More often it resides in the emotional realm, in feelings of grief, abandonment, or unexpressed pain. Buddhist teachings speak of a sea of human tears greater than the waters of the four great oceans.[4] Through meditative attention in poses of deep rest and surrender, the heart naturally opens to healing.

A Growing Legacy

In the early 2000s Judith Hanson Lasater began formally training yoga teachers in Restorative Yoga, offering workshops across the United States and Britain. Today her daughter, Lizzie Lasater, works alongside her to expand the practice, teaching globally through their online platform. Over the years Restorative Yoga has blossomed into a worldwide movement, offering a transformative path to healing, resilience, and inner peace amid the demands of an increasingly fast-paced world.

The Hidden Epidemic of Stress

Restorative Yoga has gained popularity as modern society offers little space for true relaxation. Under capitalism, productivity is prioritized over rest, and taking time to relax is frequently seen as unproductive or even lazy. In our pursuit of efficiency, we have elevated the intellect at the expense of the body and emotions, creating an imbalance that affects our well-being. Technology, originally designed to simplify our lives, has paradoxically amplified stress. Everything moves faster; everything demands immediate attention. Moments of respite have become increasingly rare. We feel an almost constant pressure to respond instantly to emails and messages or to remain perpetually updated on world events.

The growing demands of daily life leave us increasingly vulnerable to the psychological shocks that punctuate our existence. Our nervous system, chronically dysregulated, has turned stress into more than just an inevitable part of life. It has made it a constant insidious presence, quietly shaping our health, emotions, and relationships. Dr. Henry Benson, in his book *The Relaxation Response*, defines stress as environmental conditions requiring behavioral adjustments.

On a physiological level, these conditions trigger the adrenal glands to release steroid hormones, setting off a cascade of changes: elevated blood pressure, accelerated heart rate, rapid respiration, increased circulation to the muscles, and a heightened metabolic state. This reaction prepares the body to respond quickly to threats, a survival mechanism known as the fight-or-flight response.

In the 1960s, Thomas H. Holmes and Richard H. Rahe, psychiatrists at the University of Washington Medical School, developed a scale to measure life's most stressful events.[5] At the top of their list were experiences such as the death of a spouse, divorce, or marital separation. Other significant stressors included imprisonment, the death of a close family member, marriage, pregnancy, gaining a new family member, or a business readjustment. Their research revealed an important insight: Change, whether perceived as good or bad, induces stress, making individuals more vulnerable to illness as the body struggles to adapt to life's ongoing demands.

TABLE 1 The Holmes and Rahe Stress Scale

EVENT	SCALE OF IMPACT
death of a spouse	100
divorce	73
marital separation	65
imprisonment	63
death of a close family member	63
personal injury or illness	53
marriage	50
dismissal from work	47
marital reconciliation	45
retirement	45
change in health of a family member	44
pregnancy	40
sexual difficulties	39
gaining a new family member	39
business readjustment	39
change in financial state	38
death of close friend	37
change to a different line of work	36

(continues)

EVENT	SCALE OF IMPACT
change in frequency of arguments	35
major mortgage	31
foreclosure of mortgage or loan	30
change in responsibilities at work	29
child leaving home	29
trouble with in-laws	29
outstanding personal achievement	28
spouse starts or stops work	26
beginning or end of school	26
trouble with a boss	23
change in working hours or conditions	20
change in residence	20
change in schools	20
change in recreation	19
change in religious activities	19
change in social activities	18
minor mortgage or loan	17
change in sleeping habits	16
change in number of family reunions	15
change in eating habits	15
vacation	13
major holiday	12
minor violation of the law	11

score over 300: at risk of illness

score of 150–199: risk of illness is moderate, reduced by 30 percent from a score of 300

score under 150: slight risk of illness

This physiological response known as fight or flight is not inherently harmful. It plays a vital role in our survival, preparing the body to face challenges or threats. It is a fundamental aspect of our physiological and psychological makeup, enabling us to respond effectively in a wide range of situations. Under normal circumstances, the body's soothing mechanisms, governed by the parasympathetic nervous system, counterbalance this response, restoring equilibrium. In cases of chronic anxiety and depression, however, this regulatory function becomes impaired. The result is the persistent activation of the fight-or-flight response—what we commonly refer to as stress.

To better understand this phenomenon, we can examine heart rate variability (HRV), a key indicator of autonomic nervous system (ANS) activity. HRV measures the variation in time between heartbeats and reflects the balance between the sympathetic nervous system, responsible for fight or flight, and the parasympathetic nervous system, responsible for rest and digest. The ANS, via the hypothalamus, continuously regulates essential functions such as heart rate, blood pressure, breathing, and digestion to maintain balance. HRV essentially gauges the heart's ability to adapt to changing conditions and respond to stimuli. Persistent stressors such as chronic anxiety, poor sleep, unhealthy diet, dysfunctional relationships, isolation, and lack of exercise can disrupt this balance, driving the fight-or-flight response into overdrive. Research has revealed strong links among anxiety, depression, and reduced HRV. Lower HRV reflects diminished vagal tone and heightened sympathetic nervous system activity, signaling a compromised ability to regulate emotions.[6] Dr. Jean Marsac, a professor of medicine and an expert on HRV, notes that reduced HRV in adults is associated with an increased risk of cardiac events, including death, and serves as a predictor of high blood pressure. Conversely, a higher HRV indicates greater nervous system flexibility, supporting better physical and mental health.

The Role of Chronic Stress and Inflammation

Modern society often perpetuates a state of chronic fight-or-flight. Research shows that psychological stress activates the immune system, triggering the production of cytokines, molecules that are involved in inflammation. Inflammation is the body's natural defense against pathogens, injuries, or toxins, designed to protect and heal. However, persistent stress causes the immune system to remain overactivated, resulting in allostatic load and chronic inflammation.

Chronic inflammation prevents the body from recovering and resting, essential processes for optimal functioning. This contributes to the rise of stress-related illnesses, including:

- autoimmune diseases such as rheumatoid arthritis and Crohn's disease
- cardiovascular diseases such as hypertension and heart disease
- neurodegenerative disorders such as Alzheimer's disease
- cancer and other chronic conditions[7]

Inflammatory agents in the bloodstream can even bypass the blood-brain barrier, leading to neuroinflammation that disrupts critical neural circuits. Edward Bullmore, a professor of psychiatry at the University of Cambridge, explores this connection in his book *The Inflamed Mind: A Radical New Approach to Depression*. Bullmore explains how inflammation can act as a pathway to depression, linking physiological and emotional health.[8]

For example, a 2014 study of fifteen thousand children in southwest England found that those with mild inflammation at age nine were significantly more likely to experience depression by age eighteen. Numerous other studies support this connection, showing that inflammation often precedes depression.[9] Patients with depression frequently exhibit elevated levels of inflammatory markers, such as cytokines and C-reactive protein.[10]

Dr. Lucile Capuron, research director at France's National Institute of Agricultural Research in Bordeaux, further explains how inflammatory markers impact the central nervous system. These markers disrupt the production of neurotransmitters:

- serotonin, known as the "happiness hormone"
- norepinephrine, which regulates attention and sleep
- dopamine, involved in motivation and reward[11]

A reduction in these neurotransmitters is a hallmark of depression, highlighting how chronic stress and inflammation intersect to affect mental health.

The Relaxation Response

Fortunately, our bodies possess a natural and innate protective mechanism against overstress, enabling us to counteract the harmful effects of the fight-or-flight response. This mechanism is governed by the parasympathetic nervous system, primarily through the vagus nerve. Often referred to as the body's superhighway, the vagus nerve is a vital communication link between the brain and the internal organs.

The Role of the Vagus Nerve

The vagus nerve is a cranial nerve that extends from the brain, passing through the soft palate, throat, and torso to the viscera, where the intestinal microbiome and the enteric nervous system reside. Known as the "second brain," the enteric nervous system is embedded in the tissues of the esophagus, stomach, small intestine, and colon. With over a hundred million nerves—more than the spinal cord—this system underscores the complexity and interconnectedness of the body.

The vagus nerve regulates essential functions throughout the body, including the heart, lungs, throat, respiratory muscles, liver, stomach, pancreas, gallbladder, spleen, kidneys, and the small and large intestines.[12] When activated, this branch of the autonomic nervous system slows the heart rate and breathing, encourages deeper breathing, redirects blood flow from the limbs to the internal organs, and supports vital processes like digestion and reproduction. In this state, the body transitions into what is called the relaxation response, designed for rest, recovery, and healing.

The Science Behind Relaxation

Remarkably, the relaxation response can often be initiated by stimulating the anterior hypothalamus, a small but powerful brain region. The fact that such a comprehensive physiological response can be triggered by one area highlights how deeply our bodies are wired for relaxation. These neural pathways exist in all of us, no matter how anxious or overstimulated we may feel.

To activate this response, it is essential to create the right conditions. Setting aside at least twenty minutes in a calm, quiet environment allows the body to transition from stress to relaxation. By staying still in a comfortable position, reducing muscular tension, quieting the mind, and slowing and deepening the breath, we establish the foundation for profound relaxation.[13] Consistent practice reinforces these pathways, cultivating a healthy mind-body connection that delivers far-reaching benefits.

Restorative Yoga: A Natural Path to Relaxation

By regularly stimulating the vagus nerve, we can counteract the harmful effects of an inappropriately triggered fight-or-flight response. Once the relaxation response is activated, the body experiences transformative benefits:

- **improved digestion**: Blood flow is redirected to digestive organs, enhancing nutrient absorption and gut health, while also supporting a balanced microbiome.
- **enhanced immune function**: The immune system is stimulated, boosting the body's defense against illness.
- **reduced chronic inflammation**: As a key modulator of immune activity, the vagus nerve helps prevent excessive inflammatory responses, lowering the risk of chronic inflammation and related conditions.

The vagus nerve's role in managing inflammation is particularly significant. By maintaining immune homeostasis, it helps prevent the body from overreacting to perceived threats, which can lead to chronic inflammatory disorders.

A study conducted at Grenoble University Hospital in France demonstrated the efficacy of vagal neurostimulation in managing autoimmune conditions such as Crohn's disease and rheumatoid arthritis, highlighting the far-reaching benefits of nervous system regulation.[14] The encouraging news is that you don't need an implantable neurostimulator to harness the power of vagus nerve activation. Regular practice of Restorative Yoga offers a natural and accessible way to stimulate this vital nerve, allowing the body to engage its intrinsic healing mechanisms.

In 2010 a landmark study led by Janice Kiecolt-Glaser examined the inflammatory and endocrine responses of fifty healthy women—twenty-five novices and twenty-five experienced Restorative Yoga practitioners—before, during, and after a Restorative Yoga session. The participants were divided into a group that engaged in the practice and another that did not. While the session significantly boosted participants' positive affect compared to the control group, the researchers did not observe immediate changes in inflammatory or endocrine markers after the session. However, when analyzing baseline levels, a notable distinction emerged. Despite similarities in age, abdominal adiposity, and cardiorespiratory fitness, the novices' interleukin-6 levels—a key pro-inflammatory cytokine—were 41 percent higher than those of experienced practitioners. Additionally, the likelihood of detecting C-reactive protein, another biomarker of inflammation, was 4.75 times greater in novices than in experts. These findings underscore the profound effects of consistent Restorative Yoga practice in training the body to regulate stress, inflammation, and overall nervous system activity.[15]

By cultivating deep relaxation, Restorative Yoga stimulates the parasympathetic nervous system, creating an internal environment conducive to healing, regeneration, and equilibrium. In this state, the body transitions from a state of stress and survival to one of rest, recovery, and resilience. With continued practice, Restorative Yoga supports not only physical health but also emotional balance, offering a powerful antidote to the demands of modern life.

TABLE 2 Fight or Flight Versus the Relaxation Response[16]

SYSTEM, PROCESS, OR EVENT	FIGHT OR FLIGHT RESPONSE	RELAXATION RESPONSE
heart rate	↑	↓
vascular resistance (diameter of arteries)	↑	↓
blood pressure	↑	↓
finger temperature	↓	↑
respiration rate	↑	↓
oxygen consumption	↑	↓
muscle tension	↑	↓
lactate production (lack of oxygen)	↑	↓
sweating	↑	↓
skin resistance	↓	↑
epinephrine	↑	↓
norepinephrine	↑	↓
plasma renin activity (PRA)	↑	↓
cortisol	↑	↓
thyroid hormone	↑	↓
blood sugar	↑	↓
pupils	dilated	constricted
eyelids	wide open	half open or closed
digestive process	↓	↑
hair	standing on end	lying flat
immune function	↓	↑
EEG brain activity	fast, activated	slow, synchronized
hemispherical laterality	left dominant	right dominant
nostril lateralization	right more open	left more open
reticular activating system	↑	↓
posterior hypothalamus activity	↑	↓
anterior hypothalamus activity	↓	↑
basal forebrain	↓	↑
solitary tract nuclei	↓	↑

CHAPTER 2

What Is Restorative Yoga?

A Definition

For many, the word *relaxation* often conjures images of chilling out: watching TV, scrolling on a mobile phone, or lounging on the couch. While your body might appear at ease, your mind and nervous system remain highly stimulated. For others, relaxation might mean taking a nap. However, sleep and relaxation are two distinct physiological states. Psychologist, sleep researcher, and yoga teacher Roger Cole explains that during non–rapid eye movement (NREM) sleep, brain waves slow down to unconsciousness while the body relaxes. But physical relaxation during sleep is often not as profound as during a true relaxation practice. Muscles can remain tense and stress hormone levels may stay elevated, even in sleep.[1]

In contrast, Restorative Yoga creates an environment where the nervous system recalibrates and the body relaxes deeply, all while the brain remains in a state of alert observation. This conscious relaxation is transformative: It facilitates the release of long-held physical, mental, and emotional tensions. During practice, EEG brain wave patterns slow compared to active wakefulness, hovering at the threshold between consciousness and unconsciousness. This awareness during relaxation unlocks profound healing and restoration.

How Does Restorative Yoga Work?

Restorative Yoga promotes relaxation and rebalances the nervous system through multiple interconnected mechanisms.

Body Positioning

While seated or standing poses often engage the sympathetic nervous system, responsible for the fight-or-flight response, Restorative Yoga incorporates gentle or moderate inverted poses, which help activate baroreceptors, specialized sensory receptors located in the carotid sinuses and aortic sinus that regulate blood pressure. In an inverted yoga pose, where the head is positioned lower than the heart, blood pressure momentarily increases, prompting baroreceptors to send nerve signals to the vasomotor center in the medulla oblongata, leading to vascular dilation and a subsequent drop in blood pressure. Additionally, these signals influence cardiac regulation by stimulating parasympathetic activity and inhibiting sympathetic activation, which slows the heart rate and reduces cardiac contraction strength. This process, known as the baroreflex, fosters a state of cardiovascular stability and relaxation. This is why poses like Viparita Karani (Legs Up the Wall Pose) are particularly relaxing (see fig. 4.24).

Use of Props

Props provide structural support, minimizing muscular tension and enhancing physical comfort, enabling the body to fully surrender to a relaxed state. This passive support encourages deeper physiological restoration.

Reduction of Sensory Stimulation

External stimuli such as bright lights, loud noises, or strong odors can activate the fight-or-flight response. Practicing in a calm, warm, and dimly lit environment helps minimize sensory input, effectively inhibiting the midbrain reticular activating system and encouraging the relaxation response.

Breath Regulation

Mouth breathing and emphasizing inhale over exhale can lead to hyperventilation and heightened stress. Restorative Yoga emphasizes nasal breathing with extended exhales, which stimulate the vagus nerve and foster relaxation.

Mechanical Stimulation of the Vagus Nerve

Gentle pressure on the eyes using an eye bag or similar prop can stimulate the vagus nerve, slow the heart rate, and deepen relaxation.[2] Research by Roger Cole highlights that the fight-or-flight response and the relaxation response are physiologically incompatible. In other words, it is impossible to feel both anxious and relaxed simultaneously.

Case Study: Restorative Yoga and Metabolic Syndrome

A 2008 study explored the effectiveness of Restorative Yoga as an intervention for underactive, overweight adults with metabolic syndrome. Metabolic syndrome is a cluster of conditions, including high blood glucose levels, low HDL ("good cholesterol"), high triglycerides, large waist circumference, and high blood pressure, which collectively increase the risk of diabetes and cardiovascular disease. Participants were randomized into two groups: one attended fifteen Restorative Yoga sessions of ninety minutes each over ten weeks, while the other was placed on a waiting list as a control. The results were promising:

- Yoga participants showed high attendance and adherence to home practice.
- 87 percent found the poses easy to perform, with all participants giving the highest satisfaction ratings.
- The yoga group experienced trends toward reduced blood pressure, increased energy, and improved well-being compared to the control group.

The study concluded that Restorative Yoga is a feasible and effective intervention for managing metabolic syndrome in overweight adults.[3] By practicing Restorative Yoga, we enhance physical health and support the parasympathetic nervous system's ability to regulate stress and emotional responses. Regular practice fosters:

- **greater self-awareness**: observing habitual patterns without judgment
- **increased compassion**: cultivating empathy for oneself and others
- **enhanced problem-solving skills**: navigating challenges with creativity and calmness
- **emotional and spiritual growth**: Restorative Yoga offers a path to profound self-discovery and inner connection.

With consistent practice, you will discover that Restorative Yoga is not only a tool for managing chronic stress but also a gateway to self-awareness, intuition, and personal growth.

Transforming Our Relationship with Time

As explored in the following chapters, Restorative Yoga offers powerful tools to address a variety of challenges. However, like any practice, its effectiveness relies on regularity and consistency. Dedicating a minimum of twenty minutes per day helps balance the nervous system, while longer sessions allow for deeper transformation and healing. The sequences in this book are designed for practice sessions lasting forty-five to sixty minutes, excluding setup and transitions. If time is limited, focus on the final pose of the sequence, Savasana (Corpse Pose), for your daily practice. Once a week, aim to complete an entire sequence. For those facing significant challenges, practicing a full sequence two to three times per week, alongside daily Savasana, can be especially beneficial.

Finding time for Restorative Yoga can be challenging in today's fast-paced world, where we often feel like we're racing against the clock. But this practice isn't about withdrawing from life or giving up activities you enjoy. It's also not about trying to be more efficient just to save time. Instead, it encourages a mindful approach to time, helping you create a daily routine that allows you to slow down and fully appreciate life.

To begin, reflect on the beliefs and behaviors shaping your perception of time. Make an inventory of your daily activities, identifying those that feel nourishing versus draining. Consider which commitments deserve your focus and which tasks you might delegate or let go of entirely. As you become more intentional with your time, you'll naturally find ways to expand your practice. Your body and mind will reap the rewards of this dedication. The best times for practice are early in the morning, on an empty stomach, or just before bedtime to encourage restful sleep. Avoid practicing right after meals as achieving deep relaxation can be more challenging during digestion. Through this process, you'll transform not only how you approach Restorative Yoga but also how you engage with time itself, opening the door to greater balance, ease, and presence in your daily life.

Creating the Ideal Practice Environment

A calm, quiet, and warm environment with minimal sensory stimulation is essential for balancing the nervous system and fostering deep relaxation. In today's world, where sensory overload has become the norm, the ability to find silence is increasingly rare. Many of us have developed a habit of manipulating our nervous systems with external stimuli like music, films, or alcohol. While these may offer temporary distraction, they do little to restore the mind and body. Incorporating a daily "sensory fast" of at least twenty minutes is now more important than ever.

This concept is beautifully encapsulated in *pratyahara*, the conscious withdrawal of the senses, which is one of the eight limbs of yoga as outlined by Patanjali. Pratyahara serves as a cornerstone of Restorative Yoga, inviting us to gently turn our awareness inward.

The Role of Pratyahara in Restorative Yoga

The primary value of pratyahara lies in its ability to control sensory input: visual, auditory, olfactory, and proprioceptive stimulation. By reducing this input, we calm the mind by inhibiting the activity of the reticular activating system (RAS), a neural network located in the brainstem just above the spinal cord. The RAS acts as a filter for information, sensations, and emotions, keeping us alert and responsive to our environment. When the RAS is subdued, the body naturally shifts into its rest-and-digest state, promoting relaxation and overall well-being.

Guided Relaxation and the Power of Silence

In the following chapters you will find guided relaxation scripts for each pose. These scripts are designed to assist teachers in guiding students through the initial five minutes of relaxation, after which silence is encouraged. The focus on silence is a key aspect of Restorative Yoga, distinguishing it from practices like Yoga Nidra.

Restorative Yoga is deeply introspective, encouraging individuals to embark on their own inner journey. If you are practicing alone, embrace the silence and focus on the sensations within your body, setting aside the need for external guidance.

Practical Tips for Creating Your Space

Before you begin your practice, take a few moments to prepare your environment:

- Switch your phone to airplane mode to avoid disturbances.
- Ensure that you will not be interrupted for the duration of your relaxation.
- Dim the lights, adjust the temperature for comfort, and consider using props to support your pose.

By cultivating an environment that minimizes distractions and sensory input, you create the conditions for your nervous system to unwind, paving the way for true restoration and inner stillness.

The Importance of Props

Props are an essential of Restorative Yoga, providing the support needed for the body to release tension and achieve deep relaxation. One of my students once compared it to playing tennis: If you want to play tennis, you need the proper equipment. Similarly, for Restorative Yoga, equipping yourself with the right props makes all the difference. The more props you use, the more fully your body can relax.

Props not only help the body feel supported and safe but also highlight areas where tension is habitually held. To release this tension, it's crucial to create an environment where the body feels completely at ease.

The Role of Props in Restorative Yoga

Using too few props can lead to excessive stretching, which is not the goal of Restorative Yoga. Unlike practices such as Yin Yoga, Restorative Yoga is not about actively stretching the fascia or muscles. Stretching involves effort, which stimulates the nervous system, while Restorative Yoga focuses on passivity, softening, and radical presence. For example, in Salamba Setu Bandhasana (Supported Bridge Pose), you may feel a slight stretch in your chest and belly, especially when you first begin. However, the intention is to create an opening rather than a stretch, allowing the body to soften naturally into the pose.

Additionally, we use the weight of blankets, bolsters, or sandbags to stimulate the fascia and the vagus nerve. For example, placing a blanket or sandbag on the navel area helps relax and hydrate the fascia. Fascia are fibrous membranes that cover various parts of the body and fill intermediate spaces. Composed of connective tissue, fascia is closely linked to the nervous system, containing ten times more sensory nerve endings than muscles. As previously mentioned, the vagus nerve acts as a two-way communication highway. When the fascia relaxes, this information is transmitted to the brain, calming the nervous system. This is why having cotton yoga blankets that typically weigh around three pounds is so beneficial.

Props You'll Need for Restorative Yoga Poses (fig. 2.1)

1–2 sticky mats

1 yoga chair

1–2 bolsters

5–8 blankets, 60 by 80 inches and weighing 3 pounds

2 yoga bricks

4 yoga blocks

1 yoga belt

1 10-pound sandbag

1 hand towel

1–3 eye bags

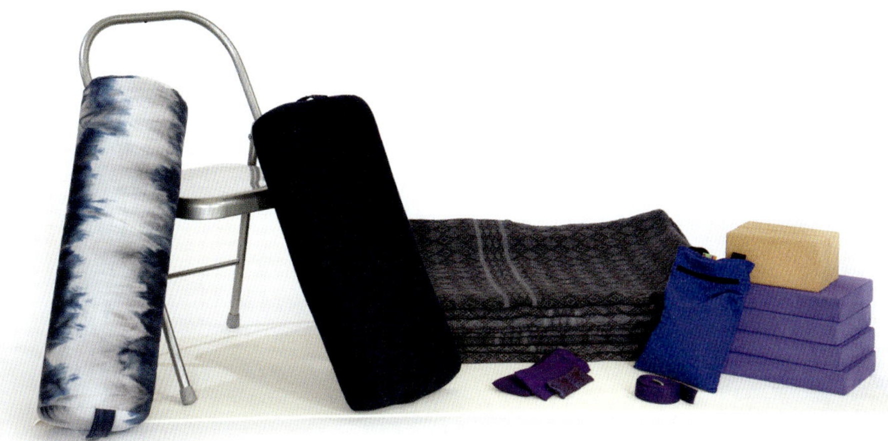

FIGURE 2.1 Basic Restorative Yoga props, including a mat, a chair, bolsters, blankets, blocks, bricks, eye pillows, a sandbag, a hand towel, and a strap.

CREATIVE ALTERNATIVES

You don't need to own every piece of equipment to get started. This book offers suggestions for creatively supporting your body using what you already have at home:

- Books can replace blocks or bricks.
- Cushions be used instead of bolsters.
- A robe belt or necktie can function as a yoga strap.
- A clean sock filled with rice can serve as an eye bag.

Having the perfect equipment isn't essential. What matters most is replicating the shape and symmetry of each pose to fully experience its benefits. Props help you adapt and personalize your practice, offering support where needed and enhancing relaxation. By customizing your setup, you create a truly restorative experience tailored to your body's unique needs.

How to Fold Your Blankets

For some, folding blankets may feel tedious at first, but it's truly an investment in your practice. A well-folded blanket can be the difference between a pose that feels merely adequate and one that you never want to leave. Blankets in Restorative Yoga are not just props; they mimic the sensation of touch, offering gentle support like an arm cradling your neck in a comforting embrace. This attention to detail allows the body to soften and relax more deeply. As you deepen your practice, you'll discover that a carefully folded blanket can transform a pose into something profoundly therapeutic. It's a small act of preparation with the potential to create a big impact on your overall experience.

TABLE 3 Five Essential Blanket Folds

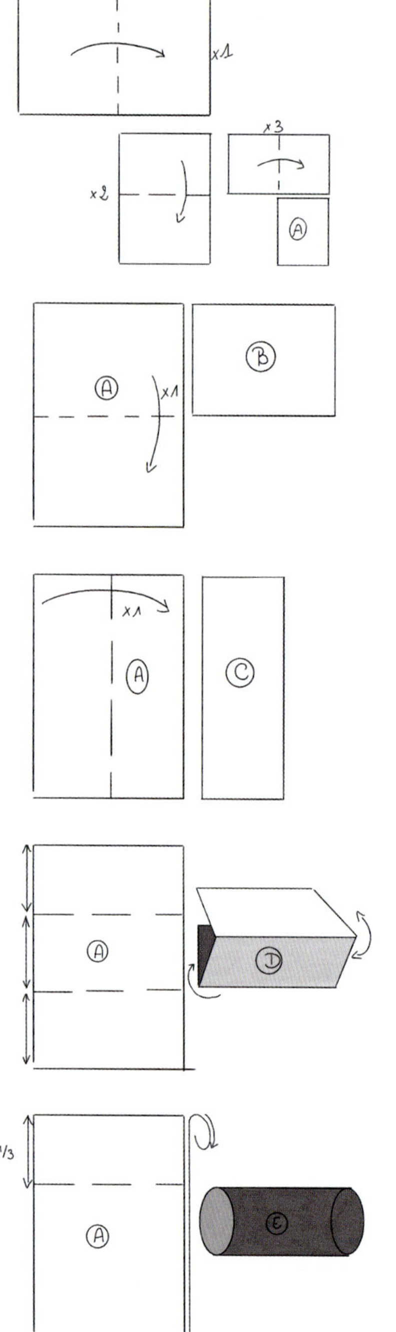

standard fold

blanket folded in half three times

size: 1 × 20 × 30 inches

single-fold square

standard fold; fold in half widthwise

size: 2 × 20 × 15 inches

single-fold rectangular

standard fold; fold in half lengthwise

size: 2 × 10 × 30 inches

double fold

standard fold; two folds widthwise

size: 3 × 20 × 10 inches

rolled blanket

standard fold; start at the short folded edge and roll the blanket

size: 5 × 6 × 20 inches

How to Support the Head, Neck, and Shoulders

The head is one of the most sensitive areas of the body during restorative practices and requires careful attention. In nearly every pose described in this book, except for certain backbends, a slight cervical flexion is preferred. This means the head is gently tipped forward, with the chin directed toward the heart. This positioning activates the parasympathetic nervous system, fostering a state of calm and relaxation.

Conversely, if the head tips backward, causing the chin to lift away from the floor and the brow to tilt upward, it can stimulate unnecessary mental activity, disrupting the relaxation process. In his book *A Physiological Handbook for Teachers of Yogasana*, Mel Robin, a physician and yoga teacher, refers to the relaxation triggered by the forward head tilt and downward gaze as the "cervical flexional reflex."[4] When the chin is slightly lowered, baroreceptors in the carotid sinuses are gently compressed, encouraging the body to lower the heart rate and blood pressure as it strives to regain homeostasis. This physiological response explains why forward bends and poses like Salamba Sarvangasana (Supported Shoulderstand, fig. 4.8) and Ardha Halasana (Half Plow Pose, fig. 4.12) are particularly soothing.

USING A BLANKET FOR OPTIMAL SUPPORT

Judith Hanson Lasater has explored how to use a blanket to effectively support the head and effectively activate this reflex. To achieve this:

- Use a standard-fold blanket (see Table 3 on page 20).
- Position the thinner edge of the blanket at the top of your shoulder blades to release tension in the shoulders.
- Fold the blanket so its thickest edge rests beneath the seventh cervical vertebra (C7), the prominent vertebra at the base of the neck, gently elevating it.
- Roll the outer edges of the blanket under, along the sides of your neck, for added stability.
- Additionally, roll the outer edges of the blanket under your outer shoulders for extra support (figs. 2.2–3).

This setup provides a stable and supported position for the head and neck, helping to prevent discomfort and even reduce the likelihood of falling asleep during the practice.

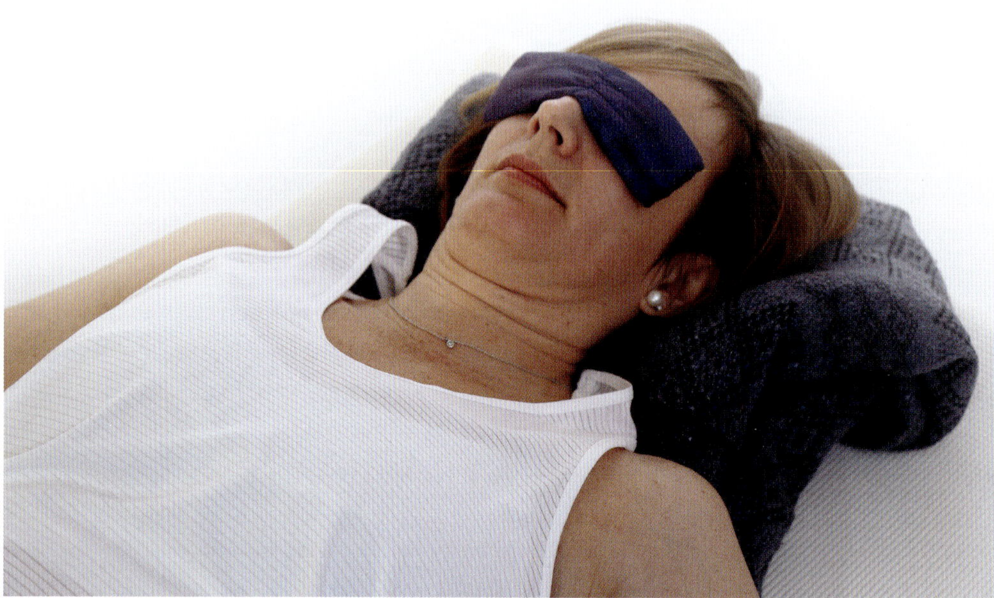

FIGURE 2.2 Audrey demonstrates Savasana with the head supported by a folded blanket and an eye pillow.

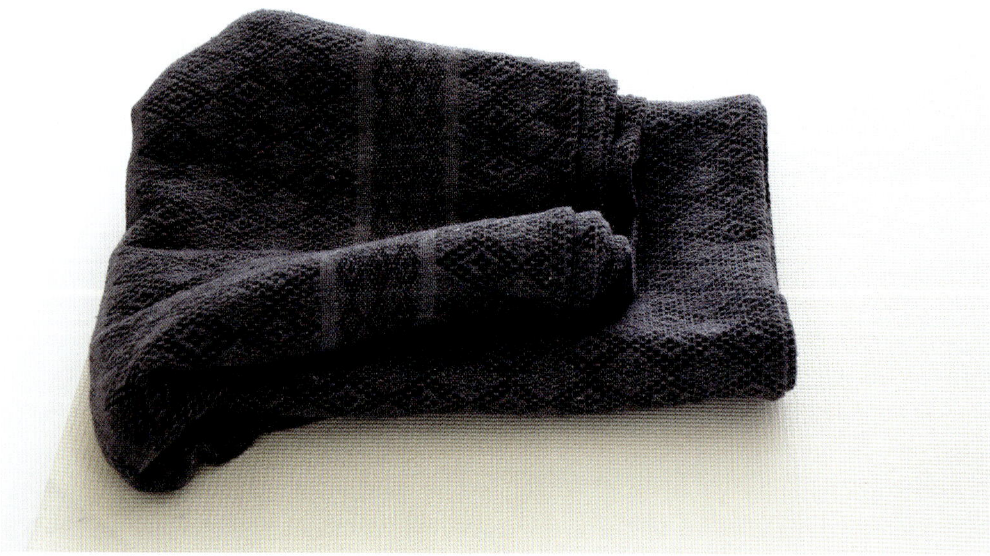

FIGURE 2.3 A yoga blanket folded to support the head and neck in Restorative Yoga poses.

ALTERNATIVE SUPPORT OPTIONS

If a blanket is unavailable, you can use a pillow to support the head and neck. Position the edge of the pillow under the top of your shoulders and the C7 vertebra. Then fold the upper corners of the pillow inward to provide a comfortable support for your head.

A Sequence of Restorative Yoga Poses

A Restorative Yoga session usually includes three to five poses, giving you enough time to fully relax in each one. Ideally, set aside sixty to ninety minutes for your practice. Move slowly and mindfully, taking your time in each pose and during transitions. Before designing a well-rounded sequence, it's important to understand that restorative poses are divided into several categories. While individual needs may vary, including poses from each category ensures a balanced practice.

Categories of Restorative Yoga Poses

PASSIVE STANDING POSES

These poses offer gentle spinal decompression and promote deep relaxation by applying light pressure on the forehead in a supported upright position. This combination helps calm the nervous system while encouraging a sense of grounding. Examples include:

- Salamba Uttanasana (fig. 3.7)
- Ardha Svanasana (fig. 4.17)
- Salamba Adho Mukha Svanasana (fig. 4.23)
- Salamba Prasarita Padottanasana (figs. 4.21–22)

45-DEGREE-ANGLE POSES

Poses practiced at a 45-degree angle help calm the nervous system while reducing the likelihood of falling asleep.[5] Examples include:

- Chaise Longue (fig. 2.5)
- Supta Baddha Konasana (fig. 4.1)
- Salamba Navasana (figs. 3.9 and 4.19)
- Salamba Supta Virasana (fig. 4.18)

BACKBENDS

Spinal extension poses such as backbends gently open the chest and support relaxation. Examples include:

- Salamba Matsyasana (fig. 2.6)
- Salamba Urdhva Dhanurasana (figs. 3.14 and 4.9)
- Salamba Setu Bandhasana (figs. 3.16–17)

These poses share some benefits of inversions but carry similar contraindications, including menstruation, pregnancy, hiatal hernia, or glaucoma.

INVERSIONS

Inversions position the head below the heart, improving blood flow to the abdominal organs, nourishing them with essential nutrients, and calming the mind. Moderate inversions include:

- Ardha Viparita Karani (fig. 3.3)
- Viparita Baddha Konasana (fig. 4.10)
- Viparita Karani (fig. 4.24)

Advanced inversions, such as Salamba Sarvangasana (fig. 4.8) and Ardha Halasana (fig. 4.12), require proper guidance to avoid injury.

TWISTS

Twists can be practiced either lying down (fig. 2.7) or seated at a 45-degree angle (fig. 3.2). Avoid ending your practice with a twist, as it creates a unilateral effect on the spine. Instead, follow twists with a forward bend or transition directly into Savasana.

FORWARD BENDS

Forward bends can be practiced seated or reclining, providing a deep sense of relaxation while gently lengthening the spine. These poses help release tension in the back and promote a calming effect on the nervous system. Examples include:

- Salamba Balasana (figs. 4.2–4)
- Salamba Upavistha Konasana (fig. 2.8)
- Adho Mukha Swastikasana (fig. 3.1)
- Salamba Janu Sirsasana (fig. 3.8)

SAVASANA VARIATIONS

Savasana is the last pose and should always end your practice. Different variations offer customized support to suit your needs.

Structuring Your Sequence

A balanced restorative sequence moves the spine in all directions without emphasizing any specific area. Always conclude with Savasana, allowing the body to integrate the physiological and mental benefits of the practice. Spending fifteen or twenty minutes in Savasana helps lower stress levels, enhance immune function, and foster a sense of calm and well-being that can last for hours. Once you've mastered the basics, you can design personalized sequences to target specific goals, such as focusing on a certain area of the body or achieving desired energetic shifts.

POSE AND COUNTERPOSE

A traditional sequencing approach pairs poses with their counterposes, for example, following a backbend with a forward bend. However, I prefer a more nuanced approach. In my experience the urge to counter a backbend with a forward bend often arises because the initial pose was too intense or unevenly compressed the spine. Instead, consider these alternatives:

- Follow a backbend with a twist such as Salamba Bharadvajasana (fig. 3.2).
- Transition to a gentler backbend such as Viparita Baddha Konasana (fig. 4.10) after Salamba Urdhva Dhanurasana with a Chair (fig. 4.9).
- Lie on your back with bent legs before moving into Savasana with Elevated Legs (fig. 4.25).

Always observe the effects of a pose before selecting the next one. If you incorporate counterposes, ensure a smooth transition with intermediate twists or gentle neutral poses.

What Kind of Breathing Should I Adopt During My Practice?

The primary goal of Restorative Yoga is to let go as deeply as possible. To support this process, practice breathing through your nose. Nasal breathing is naturally deeper and more efficient than mouth breathing. It also tends to elongate the exhale relative to the inhale, which helps lower the heart rate and calm the nervous system. Over time, as you relax more deeply, your breath will begin to regain its natural rhythm and intelligence. The tensions that once restricted your breathing will gradually fade, allowing your breath to become fuller, slower, and more profound.

Understanding Pranayama

The word *pranayama* is composed of two parts:

- *prana*: breath, respiration, or vitality
- *ayama*: without restriction

Together, *pranayama* means "breathing without restriction." When we slow and deepen our breath, the parasympathetic nervous system, responsible for the rest-and-digest state, becomes dominant. In contrast, shallow breathing triggers the sympathetic nervous system, placing the body in a state of hyperarousal.

Rapid shallow breathing, common in modern life, disrupts the body's ability to process emotions and stress. It reduces oxygen delivery to the brain, muscles, and tissues, constricts blood vessels, and over time may contribute to chronic conditions like heart disease, stroke, and other illnesses. Breathing fully and deeply is essential for emotional balance, mental clarity, and overall well-being.

Pranayama Techniques for Restorative Yoga

In poses where the chest is slightly open, such as Chaise Longue, Supta Baddha Konasana, or Savasana for Pranayama, you can focus on specific breathing techniques to regulate your breath:

- **Sama Vritti (Equal Breathing)**: Balance the inhale and exhale to the same length.
- **Visama Vritti (Unequal Breathing)**: Extend the exhale to twice as long as the inhale.
- **Bhramari (Bee's Breath)**: Produce a gentle humming sound during exhalation to soothe the nervous system.

Keep in mind that the goal of pranayama is not to breathe more but to breathe more slowly. Avoid forcing your breath or exceeding 50–60 percent of your full capacity to inhale and exhale, as overexertion can overstimulate the nervous system.

Choosing the Right Breathing Pattern

To decide which pranayama technique suits your needs, take a moment to assess your current mental state (see "Mindful Check-In" on page 47):

- If your thoughts feel slow, sluggish, or focused on the past, choose Sama Vritti to harmonize your inhale and exhale, creating balance and energy.
- If your thoughts are racing, worried, and focused on the future, opt for Visama Vritti (see "Practicing Visama Vritti (Unequal Breathing)" in chapter 3) or Bhramari (see "Bhramari Pranayama (Bee's Breath)" in chapter 3) to elongate your exhale, slow your heart rate, and soothe your nervous system.

These techniques help regulate your emotions, calm your mind, and bring you into a state of equilibrium.

A Note on Safety

You're now ready to begin! But always prioritize your safety: If you experience any discomfort, pain, or uncertainty during your practice, pause immediately and consult a health care professional. Restorative Yoga is meant to support your journey toward relaxation and healing. Listen to your body and approach your practice with care and mindfulness.

A Balanced Sequence for Your Daily Practice

This sequence is designed to move your spine in all directions while stimulating the functioning of your abdominal organs. In traditional yoga teachings, the health of these organs is considered fundamental to overall well-being. The poses in this sequence aim to enhance blood circulation in and around these organs through a technique referred to as "squeezing and soaking."

The Squeezing and Soaking Technique

This approach involves two complementary actions.

- **Soaking**: Certain poses increase blood flow to the abdominal organs, bathing them in oxygen and nutrients to support optimal function.
- **Squeezing**: Other poses gently compress the abdominal area, encouraging the release of stagnant fluids and promoting detoxification.[6]

By integrating these complementary actions, this sequence not only nourishes your abdominal organs but also supports improved digestion, detoxification, and a sense of overall vitality.

Chaise Longue Pose

10–15 MINUTES

Chaise Longue is a rejuvenating pose that gently removes the barriers restricting our full breathing capacity. By surrendering to the support of the ground and props, the body can release deeply held tension in the abdomen and rib cage.

As the body softens and unwinds, the breath begins to flow more freely, gradually deepening in a natural and unforced way. Over time, this practice cultivates a sense of ease and expansion in the breath, promoting a profound state of relaxation and renewal.

PROPS NEEDED

1 mat, 6 blocks, 1 brick, 2 bolsters, 4 blankets, 1 eye bag

SETTING UP THE POSE

- Start by placing two blocks lengthwise on your yoga mat, stacked one on top of the other. Add a brick horizontally on top of the blocks. Then position a bolster lengthwise on top of the brick. The goal is to create a 45-degree angle.
- Cover the bolster and the floor with a blanket folded in half widthwise to provide extra comfort for your back (fig. 2.4).
- At the top of the bolster, add a standard-fold blanket folded into two layers. The higher layer should support your head, with the thickest edge placed under the C7 vertebra for optimal support. The lower layer, with its thinnest edge, supports the top of your shoulder blades.

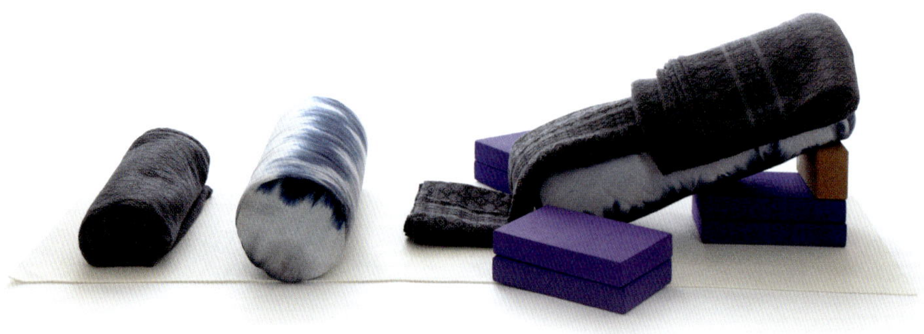

FIGURE 2.4 Setup for Chaise Longue Pose using blocks, bolsters, and folded blankets to support the back and legs while encouraging gentle chest opening.

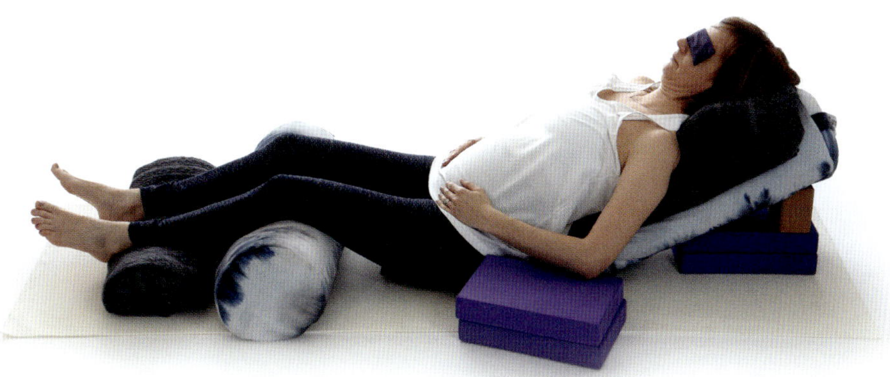

FIGURE 2.5 Audrey demonstrates Chaise Longue Pose, with full support under the back and legs to promote chest opening and relaxation.

- Sit in front of the bolster with your legs extended in front of you. Lie back onto the bolster. Ensure there is no gap between your pelvis and the bolster to ensure optimal lumbar support and help open your sternal area.
- Bend your knees and place a second bolster under them. Position a rolled blanket under your Achilles tendons. For optimal comfort, the support under your knees should be approximately twice the height of the blanket beneath your ankles.
- Adjust the blanket under your head, rolling its outer edges along the sides of your neck, your head, and your outer shoulders to provide complete support.
- Rest your hands gently on your abdomen and support your elbows with two blocks on each side of your body (fig. 2.5).
- Cover yourself with a blanket, place an eye bag over your eyes, and relax for 10–15 minutes in silence and dim lighting to calm your nervous system and mind.

If You Feel Discomfort in Your Lower Back

- Place an additional standard-fold blanket under your seat to reduce the arch from floor to bolster.

GUIDING STUDENTS THROUGH RELAXATION

During the practice, you can use the following guidance to help students relax deeply and connect with the pose:

- Begin by taking a few deep breaths through your nose, noticing all the places where your body meets the ground and the props.

- Bring your attention to your hands. With each exhale, allow your fingers to relax. Feel your arms grow heavy, your shoulders soften, and your legs rest more deeply.
- Shift your awareness to your spine. With each exhale, release all areas of tension, letting your spine gently settle onto the bolster. Feel the back of your head relaxing into the blanket, and let this wave of calm gently envelop your face. Smooth the skin of your forehead outward toward your temples. Focus on the area between your eyebrows, releasing any tension there. Relax the outer muscles of your jaw and the root of your tongue, allowing them to soften completely. Take a moment to notice the profound sense of peace that now radiates across your face.
- Let this wave of relaxation flow into your neck and throat, then down into your belly and around your navel. Imagine this feeling of ease reaching deep into your abdomen, softening even the muscles you cannot see but you can imagine.
- With every exhale, allow the weight of your body to sink farther into the props, as though you are floating effortlessly on the surface of a still lake. Now imagine yourself gently slipping below the surface, surrounded by a world of quiet and calm, with the water holding you tenderly. Whatever thoughts or feelings arise, let them drift away like leaves carried by a gentle current. Continue to let go, sinking deeper and deeper into stillness and silence.

TRANSITIONING OUT OF THE POSE

- As your relaxation draws to a close, reconnect with the space around you by taking slow, deep breaths. If you feel the need, allow yourself to yawn.
- Move at your own pace, starting with small movements in your fingers and toes.
- Slowly turn your knees inward.
- Inhale, and as you exhale, press your lower back gently against the bolster.
- Take another deep breath in, and on the exhale, bend one knee, then the other, placing your feet on the bolster.
- Inhale, and as you exhale, roll onto the side of the bolster, letting your eye bag softly fall to the floor.
- When you feel ready, use an exhale to slowly return to a seated position, supporting yourself with your hands.

Salamba Matsyasana (Supported Fish Pose)

8–10 MINUTES

Salamba Matsyasana, or Supported Fish Pose, is a powerful antidote to the effects of prolonged sitting, an all too common aspect of modern life. By gently opening the chest and elongating the spine, this pose encourages deeper breathing, reduces fatigue, and promotes a sense of rejuvenation.

The heart-opening quality of this asana helps relieve tension in the shoulders and upper back, promoting a feeling of lightness and ease. Additionally, this pose enhances circulation to the abdominal organs, delivering oxygen and vital nutrients to support optimal digestion and overall well-being.

CONTRAINDICATIONS

- pregnancy beyond the third trimester
- sinusitis or cold
- gastroesophageal reflux
- spondylolysis and spondylolisthesis
- glaucoma or other conditions requiring care with intraocular pressure

PROPS NEEDED

1 mat, 1 bolster, 4 blankets, 1 eye bag

SETTING UP THE POSE

- Take a standard-fold blanket and unfold it lengthwise across the middle of your mat. Fold it accordion-style across its width to create four even waves. This will provide the central lift needed to open the chest and support the diaphragm.
- Unfold a second standard-fold blanket lengthwise and position it at the top of the mat. Roll its lower edge tightly to form a little cushion that supports the tops of your shoulders and the C7 vertebra. Ensure the roll is firm yet comfortable. It should not go under the skull or cervical spine.
- Sit on your mat just in front of the accordion-folded blanket, then slowly recline, allowing your thoracic spine to settle onto the folds so they support the area just below your shoulder blades. This positioning gently lifts the root of your diaphragm, located near the T11 and T12 thoracic vertebrae, encouraging a soft, spacious opening through the upper abdomen. Ensure that both your pelvis and your lower back remain unsupported.

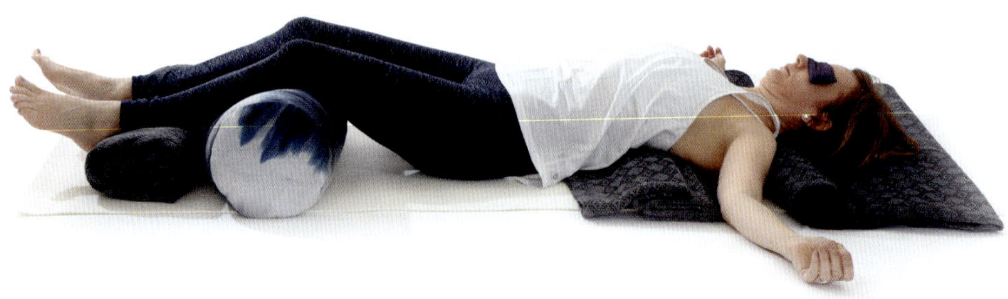

FIGURE 2.6 Audrey demonstrates Salamba Matsyasana with props under the chest, C7, knees, and ankles, and an eye pillow to encourage deep relaxation.

- If you feel tension when swallowing, or tightness in the jaw or throat, your roll is too high, near the skull. Readjust to lift the C7 vertebra slightly forward and then let the head release back.
- Place a bolster under your knees to help ease tension in your lower back, and position a rolled blanket beneath your Achilles tendons for added support. Ideally, your knees should be elevated to about twice the height of your ankles. This gentle incline encourages the thigh bones to settle into the hip sockets, allowing the lower spine to release and the entire back of the body to relax more fully into the ground.
- Rest your arms along your sides, slightly away from your body, at about a 90-degree angle. This position encourages the chest to open naturally and supports fuller, more easeful breathing (fig. 2.6).
- Cover yourself with a blanket to maintain warmth and comfort.
- Close your eyes and place an eye pillow gently over them to encourage relaxation and block out light.
- Stay in this pose for 8–10 minutes. Use a soft timer to gently signal the end of your practice.

GUIDING STUDENTS THROUGH RELAXATION

During the practice, you can use the following guidance to help students relax deeply and connect with the pose:

- Begin by breathing naturally through your nose. Let your jaw relax, your lips soften, and your tongue settle effortlessly in your mouth. Feel your face become serene, as if a gentle wave of relaxation is washing over it.

- Slowly bring your awareness to your body. Begin a gentle body scan, starting from your heels and moving upward to the crown of your head. At each point of contact with the floor or props, allow the full weight of your body to release into the support.
- Start with your heels. As you exhale, feel the weight of your feet dropping heavily into the blanket. Notice how your lower legs are cradled by the props.
- Now shift your attention to your pelvis and lower belly. With each exhale, let this area release tension, sinking naturally into the floor. Picture your belly softening like a calm pool of water, spreading gently and effortlessly into the earth.
- Bring your focus to your upper back. Feel it broadening across the blanket, your shoulder blades gently settling and spreading wide. Allow your arms and hands to rest at ease, their weight sinking effortlessly into the ground. Notice the heaviness of your head, fully supported and cradled gently by the ground.
- Shift your awareness to your heart center and chest. With each inhale, feel your breath expand and lift the upper chest, creating a sense of lightness. As you exhale, sense your upper back spreading even wider across the blanket, grounding you more deeply. Visualize your breath as a gentle wave. Imagine inhaling through the front of your chest, filling the heart, and exhaling softly through the back, releasing tension into the earth.
- Let your breath flow freely, gently softening everything it touches. As your upper back becomes more grounded, notice a natural opening in your throat. Notice a sense of ease and openness here, as if your breath flows effortlessly through this space.
- Imagine the roof of your mouth softening and widening, creating a sense of expansion. Let this spaciousness extend to the sides of your mouth, toward your teeth, and even to the base of your jaw, cultivating a feeling of openness and freedom throughout your entire face.
- Now envision a gentle stream of energy, like a clear cascading brook. This revitalizing flow begins at the soles of your feet, gently moving upward. Feel it pooling in your belly, streaming through your heart, cleansing your chest, and flowing gently through your throat. It continues upward, flowing out through the crown of your head, leaving a sense of clarity and renewal in its wake. Imagine this stream washing away tension, carrying it effortlessly out of your body, and replacing it with a refreshing sense of calm and vitality.

- Rest here for a few moments. Feel yourself fully supported by the ground. Let your breath maintain its soothing, gentle rhythm. Imagine the earth holding you gently, like a warm and steady embrace.

TRANSITIONING OUT OF THE POSE

- When it is time to come out of the pose, gently bring your awareness to the sensations of contact with the ground and the props supporting you.
- Slowly turn your knees inward.
- Bring your lower back down toward the floor.
- Bend one knee, then the other, and rest your feet on the bolster.
- Roll to your side, letting your eye bag fall gently to the floor.
- When you are ready, take your time to sit up, using your hands to support yourself as you come back to a seated position.

Salamba Jathara Parivartanasana (Supported Supine Twist)

3–4 MINUTES EACH SIDE

Jathara Parivartanasana combines the Sanskrit words *jathara*, meaning abdomen, and *parivartana*, meaning turning or rotating. In this asana, the abdomen undergoes a gentle internal massage, stimulating the optimal functioning of key organs, including the liver, stomach, pancreas, and spleen. This pose also enhances respiratory health by stretching the intercostal muscles, expanding the capacity for deeper breathing, and promoting an overall sense of vitality and well-being.

By integrating elements of a spinal twist, a backbend, and an inversion, Jathara Parivartanasana provides comprehensive benefits, offering relief from lower-back discomfort while nurturing balance and harmony in the body.

CONTRAINDICATIONS

- hiatal hernia
- pregnancy
- menstruation
- sinusitis or cold
- gastroesophageal reflux
- glaucoma or other conditions requiring care with intraocular pressure

PROPS NEEDED

1 mat, 1–2 rectangular bolsters, 3–5 blankets, 1 small towel, 1 eye bag

SETTING UP THE POSE

- Place a bolster horizontally in the middle of your mat. To increase its height, you can add a single-fold rectangular blanket on top of the bolster.
- Sit on the mat next to the long side of the bolster, positioning yourself in the center. Bend your knees and place your feet on the floor.
- Slowly lie back on your left side so that your diaphragm rests in the center of the bolster and your shoulders lightly touch the floor.
- Make sure you are lying exactly on your side, with your body rolling neither forward nor backward.
- Rest the left side of your face on a double-fold blanket for comfort and elevation. If desired, add a small rolled towel under your neck for additional support and relaxation.

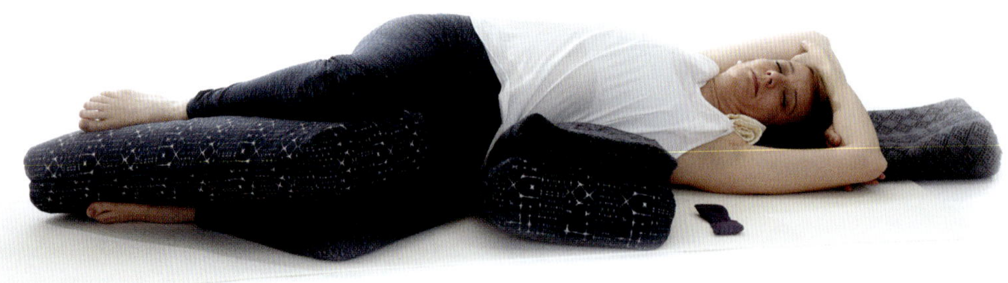

FIGURE 2.7 Audrey demonstrates Salamba Jathara Parivartanasana with bolsters for leg and torso support and a folded blanket under the head to facilitate gentle spinal rotation.

- Bring your knees toward your chest until your thighs form a 90- to 110-degree angle with your torso. Place a rectangular bolster or two single-fold rectangular blankets between your knees to keep them supported and aligned.
- Slowly raise your arms overhead. Bend them gently and use your left hand to hold your right arm just above the elbow. Apply a gentle pull on your right arm to create a stretch along the side of your torso, opening the intercostal muscles and flaring your ribs.
- Cover your entire body with a blanket to stay warm and relaxed during the pose.
- Gradually initiate a twist to the right by gently moving your right shoulder blade toward the mat. Keep your knees and feet together as you twist. Find balance in the movement, allowing your knees to gently fall to the side while you feel an opening in your right shoulder and side body. The movement should feel effortless and soothing (fig. 2.7).
- Allow your eyes to close softly if you feel comfortable. Place an eye pillow over them to encourage deeper relaxation and block out light.

GUIDING STUDENTS THROUGH RELAXATION

During the practice, you can use the following guidance to help students relax deeply and connect with the pose:

- Begin by bringing your awareness to the inner lining of your rib cage. With each inhale, feel your ribs gently expand, creating space from within. Notice how your right ribs open from hip to armpit, stretching effortlessly. As you exhale, sense the ribs gently drawing back toward your spine, like a soft wave retreating to the shore. Imagine each breath cleansing the rib cage, releasing tension and dissolving any resistance.

Each inhale washes through your ribs, while each exhale softens and melts away tightness.

- Shift your attention to your pelvis, especially the top hip. Visualize your breath flowing through this space like a gentle stream, creating openness. With every exhale, feel the weight of your hips sinking deeper into the support, grounding you with each breath.
- Let your breath flow freely through the entire inner pelvis. With each inhale, imagine a soft expansion, a sense of spaciousness. With every exhale, allow any lingering tension to dissolve, leaving your pelvis relaxed and at ease.
- Now bring your focus to your mid–rib cage, waistline, and lower ribs. Feel your breath expanding this area, widening and lengthening the side body with each inhale. With every exhale, settle your awareness here, noticing how your breath creates a gentle rhythm of expansion and release.
- Gradually guide your attention upward, traveling from the waistline into the upper torso. Feel your breath spreading through the rib cage, flowing into the armpit, and filling the shoulder. Each inhale brings lightness and freedom, as if your breath could lift away any heaviness. With each exhale, let everything settle downward, grounding your body further into deep relaxation.
- Stay here for a few moments, letting your breath naturally soothe and restore your body. Visualize the entire side body, from hip to shoulder, bathed in calm, spacious energy.
- When you feel ready, gently release the twist. Slowly align your torso parallel to your pelvis, moving with care and mindfulness. Take your time as you bring your right arm back alongside your body.
- Place your right hand on the floor in front of you and press gently into the ground to return to a seated position. Move slowly and deliberately, pausing for a moment in your seated pose to observe the effects of the twist.
- Before transitioning to the other side, take a few breaths to feel the spaciousness and ease created in your body. When you're ready, set up for the pose on the opposite side.

TRANSITIONING OUT OF THE POSE

- After completing the pose on both sides, release the twist and slowly bring your torso parallel to your pelvis. Take your time as you bring your left arm back alongside your body.
- Place your left hand on the floor in front of you and press gently into the floor to return to a seated position and observe the effects of the twist.

Salamba Upavistha Konasana (Supported Wide-Angle Seated Forward Bend)

3–5 MINUTES

This position gently stimulates blood circulation in the pelvic region, supporting the regulation of menstrual flow and promoting ovarian health. This pose not only nurtures the physical body but also encourages mental stillness. The soft pressure of the chair on the forehead activates the parasympathetic nervous system, helping to quiet the mind and slow the flow of thoughts. This combination of physical and mental benefits makes it soothing and rejuvenating.

CONTRAINDICATION

- disc disease

PROPS NEEDED

1 mat, 1 chair, 4–7 blankets, 1 eye pillow

SETTING UP THE POSE

- Place a chair at one end of your yoga mat with the seat facing you. Position a single-fold square blanket on the chair seat for added padding and comfort.
- Sit facing the chair on the corner of one or more single-fold square blankets. Elevating your pelvis helps tilt it slightly forward, creating a gentle lumbar curve and promoting length in your spine. Adjust the height to ensure your hips are slightly higher than your thighs so you can lean forward without strain.
- Extend your legs into a wide V shape, keeping them symmetrically aligned with the axis of your torso. Avoid overextending to prevent strain on your inner knees. If you feel discomfort, bring your legs closer together. Remember, the goal of Restorative Yoga is not to stretch but to create space and openness.
- To support your knees and maintain proper alignment, place two rolled blankets along the side of each leg. These props help keep your knees and toes pointing upward and reduce tension in your inner thighs.
- Slowly lean forward, cross your arms, and rest them on the chair seat in front of you. Adjust the distance from the chair so that you can maintain an extended lower back while remaining comfortable.

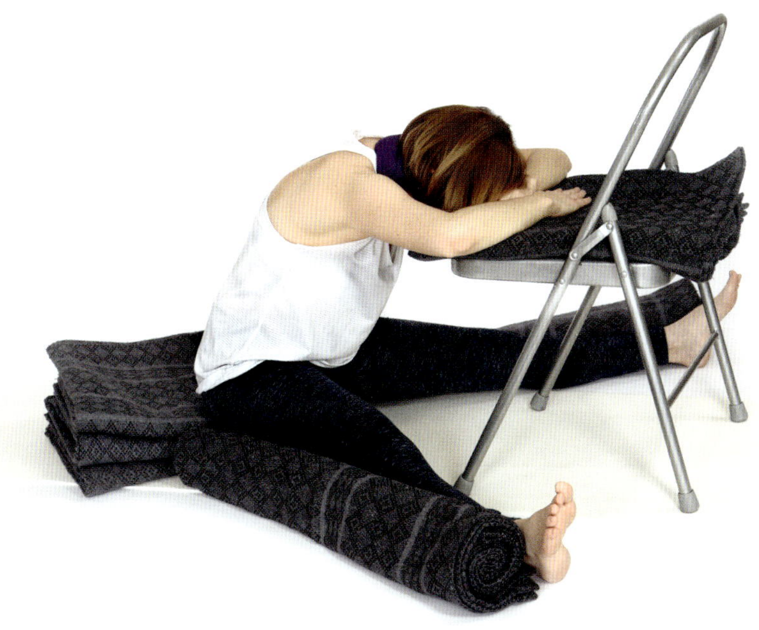

FIGURE 2.8 Audrey demonstrates Salamba Upavistha Konasana, seated on the corner of the three blankets to encourage pelvic tilt, and rolled blankets against the legs for comfort and release.

- Rest your forehead on the blanket placed on the chair seat. Alternatively, turn your head to one side, switching sides midway through the pose to balance the stretch (fig. 2.8).
- Ensure your neck does not collapse when placing your forehead on the chair. If you feel any strain in your neck, add an additional blanket to the chair seat to bring the support closer to your head.
- Cover yourself with a blanket to stay warm and relaxed. Place an eye pillow at the back of your neck to encourage deeper relaxation. Close your eyes and allow the props and pose to fully support you. Adjust your position or props if any part of your body feels tense or unsupported.

GUIDING STUDENTS THROUGH RELAXATION

During the practice, you can use the following guidance to help students relax deeply and connect with the pose:

- Allow yourself to settle into stillness. Begin to observe your breath. Inhale and exhale through your nose, allowing your breath to flow naturally, like a gentle tide flowing in and out.

- Soften your eyes, your face, your head, and your neck completely. With each breath, feel a gentle wave of ease cascading through your body, washing away any tension. Notice how your facial muscles release, your jaw unclenches, and your entire head becomes light and free.
- Bring your awareness to your hands. As you exhale, imagine all tension melting away from your fingers, palms, and wrists, leaving them soft and light, as though they could float. Feel the sensation of ease spreading up through your arms.
- Shift your focus to your abdomen. Allow your breath to flow deeply into this space, expanding gently on the inhale and releasing fully on the exhale. Picture your abdomen softening, like a pool of water rippling calmly, sending soothing waves throughout your body. With each breath, invite a deeper sense of softness and release.
- Gradually, bring your attention to your thighs. Feel the weight of your legs resting naturally on the blankets. Allow the muscles of your thighs to relax completely. Sense how the support of the blankets holds you, creating a feeling of being cradled and secure.
- Rest in the stillness of this moment, poised between the open feeling in your belly and hips, and the quiet stillness in your chest, eyes, and brain. Let your breath guide you deeper into this balance, as if your body is effortlessly suspended in a calm, timeless space.
- With each exhale, let go of anything unnecessary. Allow yourself to simply be—at ease, supported, and fully present.

TRANSITIONING OUT OF THE POSE

- When it is time to come out of the pose, open your eyes, and when you feel ready, uncross your arms and use your hands to gently press yourself back to an upright seated position.
- Bring your legs together slowly, bending them slightly if needed.
- Sit upright for a few moments to allow your body to adjust before moving to your next pose.

Salamba Savasana (Supported Corpse Pose)

20 MINUTES

"Lying flat on the ground like a corpse is called Savasana. This removes fatigue and gives rest to the mind."[7] Savasana (Corpse Pose) is a cornerstone relaxation pose in Restorative Yoga. It gently directs your energy inward, soothing the nervous system and reducing physiological stress markers. By promoting a state of deep rest, it enhances digestion, strengthens the immune system, and supports overall reproductive health.

When held for approximately twenty minutes, Salamba Savasana allows both the body and the mind to experience profound stillness, cultivating a sense of inner tranquility. It invites you to surrender completely, a conscious letting go, akin to embracing death while remaining vibrantly alive.

Also known as Mrtasana, this pose symbolizes the physical body as a lifeless form while the soul continues to radiate in a state of pure awareness. It offers a unique opportunity to explore the subtle layers of your being, connecting presence with surrender and renewal.

CONTRAINDICATION

After the first trimester of pregnancy, it is recommended to practice Side-Lying Savasana on your left side (fig. 4.20). Lying flat on your back is not advised during this stage, as it can compress the vena cava, a major blood vessel, potentially restricting blood flow to the heart and the baby. Side-Lying Savasana on the left side ensures optimal circulation and provides greater comfort and safety for both the pregnant practitioner and the baby.

PROPS NEEDED

1 mat, 1 bolster, 5 blankets, 1 eye pillow

SETTING UP THE POSE

- Sit on your mat with your knees bent in front of you and your feet flat on the floor. Cover your legs with a blanket for warmth and comfort.
- Fold a standard blanket into two layers and place it horizontally at the top of your mat. The higher layer should support your head, with the thickest edge placed under the C7 vertebra for optimal support, while the lower layer, with its thinnest edge, supports the top of your shoulder blades. Roll the blanket's edges gently to cradle the sides of your neck, head, and outer shoulders for full support.
- Place a bolster under your knees, ensuring your kneecaps rest at its center. Add a rolled blanket under your Achilles tendons to relieve tension.

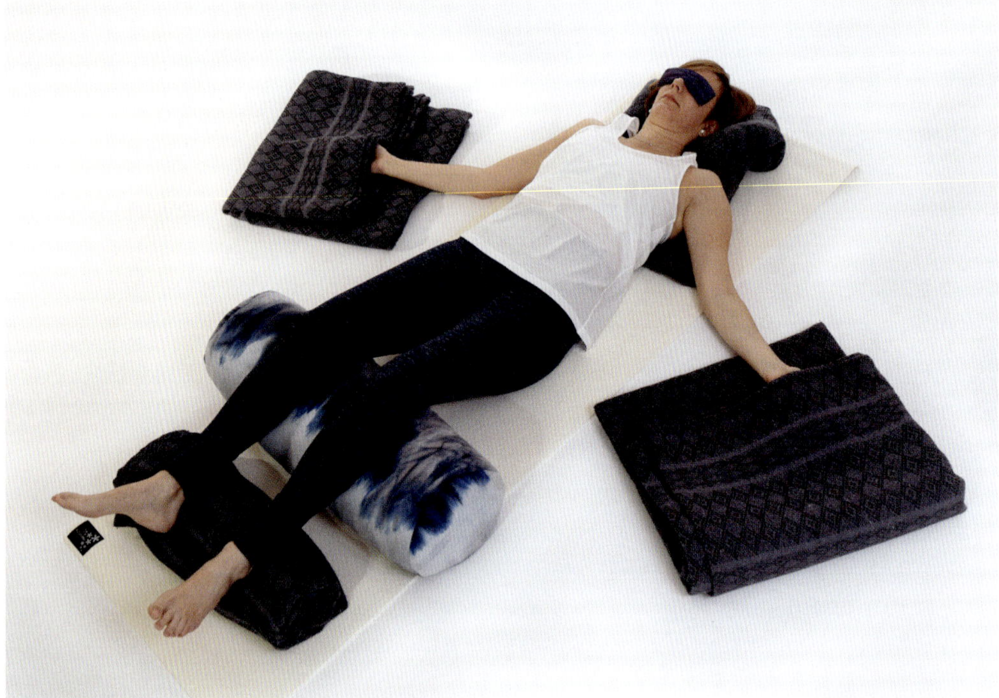

FIGURE 2.9 Audrey demonstrates fully supported Salamba Savasana with props under the head, knees, ankles, and hands to promote complete release and ease.

- Lie back comfortably, allowing your arms to rest at a minimum 45-degree angle from your torso. Let your elbows relax on the ground with your palms gently facing upward. You may place your forearms and hands on single-fold square blankets positioned on either side of your body. Your wrists should rest on the second fold of the blanket, with an additional blanket layer draped over your hands for a gentle comforting touch (fig. 2.9).
- Gently release the back of your head, inviting a sense of calm and mental stillness.
- Cover your body with a blanket for warmth and place a small eye pillow over your eyes to soften the light and promote relaxation.
- Allow your body to relax and stay in this position for twenty minutes.

GUIDING STUDENTS THROUGH RELAXATION

During the practice, you can use the following guidance to help students relax deeply and connect with the pose:

- Begin Savasana by observing your muscles gradually softening, your breath slowing, and your body releasing tension. This initial stage focuses on physiological relaxation, which may take about 15 minutes, depending on your ability to let go.

- As deep relaxation settles in, you may feel yourself gently withdrawing from the external world while maintaining subtle awareness of it. In this state, external stimuli no longer disturb your body or mind.
- This state of nonreaction is known as pratyahara, the practice of withdrawing the senses. Through pratyahara, we learn to respond less intensely to painful experiences, negative thoughts, and emotions. With practice, we gain the ability to choose our response: to engage with a stimulus or to step back and observe without reacting.
- Savasana offers a space to cultivate this inner calm. In the midst of emotional chaos, we can consciously choose not to react, conserving our energy and grounding ourselves. This practice empowers us to remain centered and resilient in the face of life's challenges.

TRANSITIONING OUT OF THE POSE

- As your practice comes to an end, begin to reconnect with the space around you by taking slow, deep breaths.
- When you feel ready, slowly turn your knees inward.
- Guide your sacrum gently down to the floor and hold it there.
- Bend one knee, then the other, and rest your feet on the bolster.
- Roll onto the side of your choice, letting your eye pillow fall softly to the floor. Stay here for at least three breaths.
- When you're ready to sit up, press the hand closest to your chest firmly into the ground, using your other hand for support. Move slowly and with intention, returning to a seated position. Take a moment to feel the transition and carry the sense of calm from your practice into the rest of your day.

Each pose has its own unique personality. Some will quickly become your favorites, while others may feel less appealing—and that's completely natural. For now, set aside the ones you find challenging or unenjoyable. Our preferences often shift with time, as our needs and experiences evolve. When you revisit these poses later, you may find yourself connecting with them in an entirely new way.

Balanced Restorative Yoga Sequences

SEQUENCE 2

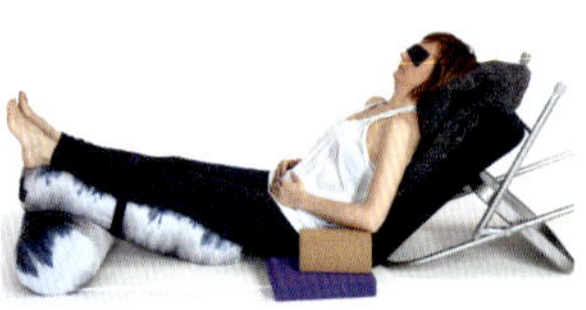

Salamba Navasana
(page 164)
10–15 minutes

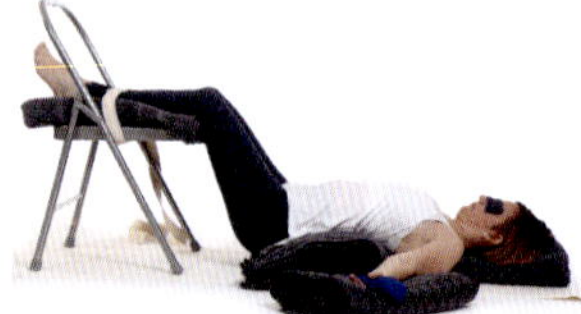

Ardha Viparita Karani
(page 56)
10–15 minutes

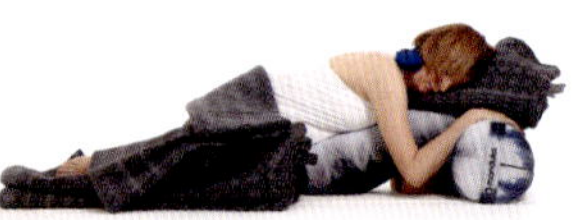

Salamba Bharadvajasana
(page 53)
2–3 minutes on each side

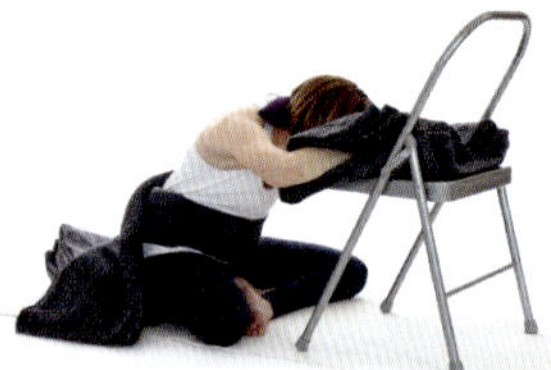

Adho Mukha Swastikasana
(page 50)
2–3 minutes

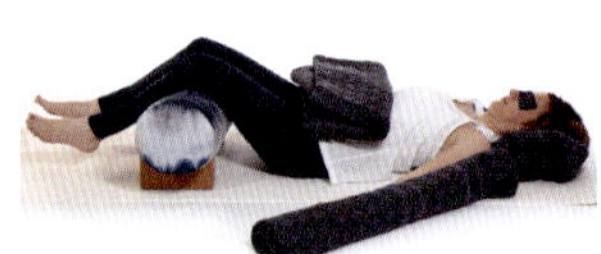

Savasana with Elevated Legs
(page 187)
20 minutes

SEQUENCE 3

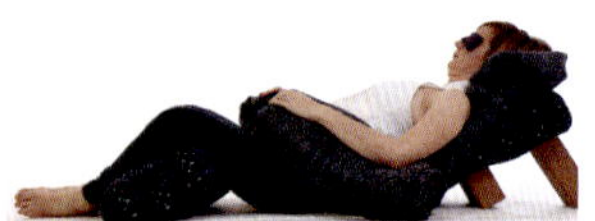

Supta Baddha Konasana
(page 113)
10–15 minutes

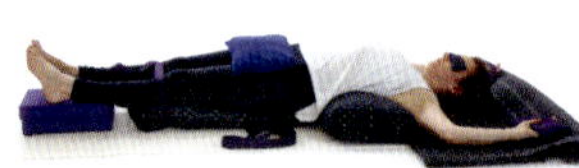

Salamba Setu Bandhasana
with Straight Legs (page 94)
8–12 minutes

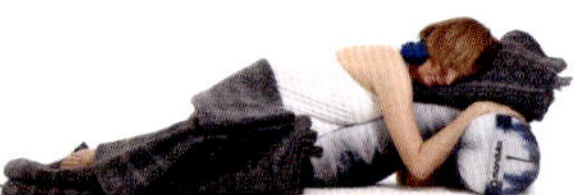

Salamba Bharadvajasana
(page 53)
2–3 minutes on each side

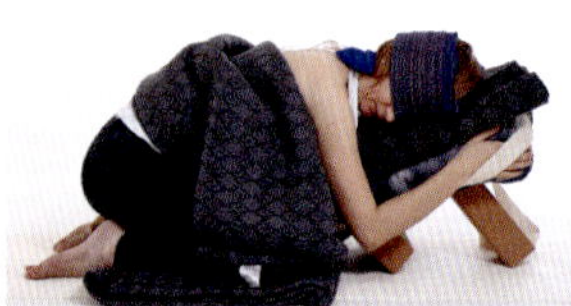

Salamba Balasana with One
Bolster (page 118)
2–3 minutes on each side

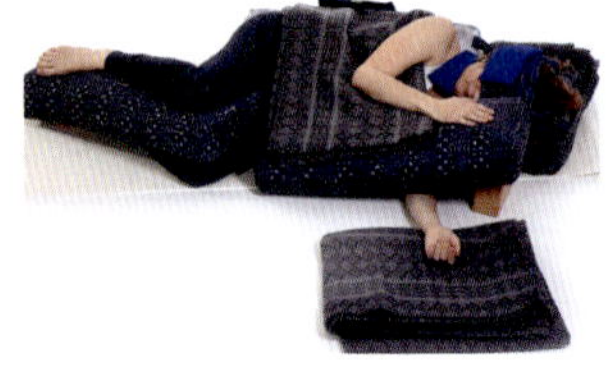

Side-Lying Savasana
(page 168)
20 minutes

SEQUENCE 4 FOR ADVANCED STUDENTS

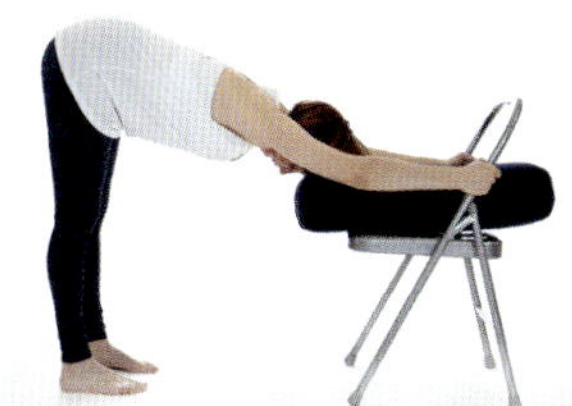

Salamba Adho Mukha Svanasana (page 180)
2–3 minutes

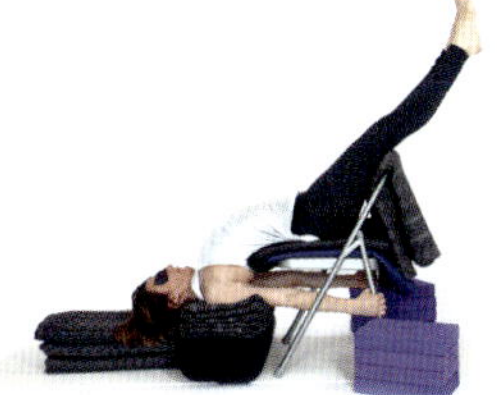

Salamba Sarvangasana (page 129)
8–15 minutes

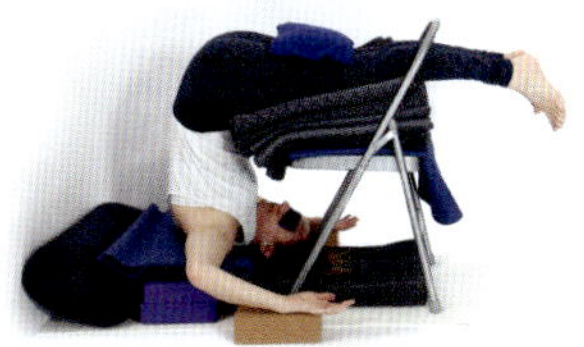

Ardha Halasana (page 141)
8–12 minutes

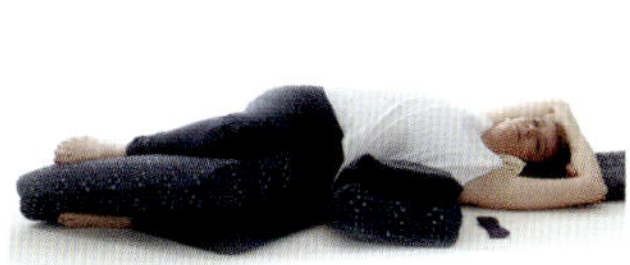

Salamba Jathara Parivartanasana (page 35)
2–3 minutes on each side

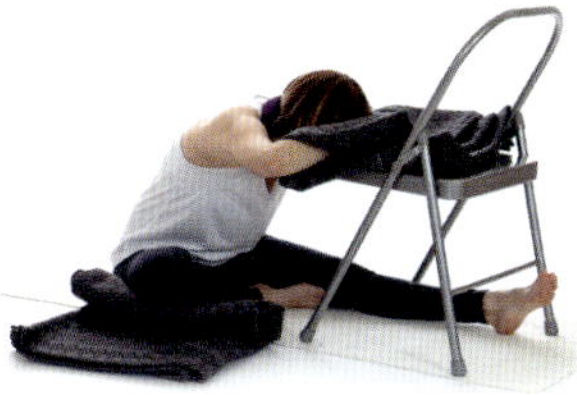

Salamba Janu Sirsasana (page 74)
2–3 minutes on each side

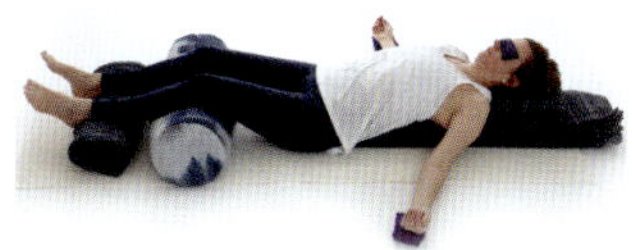

Savasana for Pranayama (page 60)
20 minutes

CHAPTER 3

Cultivating Emotional Balance

Cultivating emotional balance empowers us to develop resilience: the ability to recover and restore equilibrium after facing negative experiences. Emotional resilience isn't about avoiding challenges or maintaining perfect calm in the midst of chaos; rather, it's about exiting the fight-or-flight response more swiftly and avoiding becoming stuck in a state of heightened stress. It begins with learning how to soothe the nervous system and quiet the mind, creating space for thoughtful, intentional responses instead of reactive patterns.

As discussed earlier, you can alternate between balanced practices and sessions that target specific emotional goals, such as addressing anxiety, anger, or depression. To discover the sequence that best supports your needs, start your practice with a mindful check-in. This simple yet transformative technique, inspired by the work of clinical psychologist and yoga teacher Bo Forbes, allows you to reconnect with yourself on a deeper level. The mindful check-in is a straightforward and powerful method for identifying physical, mental, and emotional tension. Its adaptability makes it easy to integrate into your daily routine, providing opportunities to pause, reflect, and reset whenever needed. With just a few moments of mindful attention, the check-in serves as a grounding practice that fosters calm and cultivates emotional balance, setting the tone for your Restorative Yoga journey.

Mindful Check-In

5 MINUTES

- **Find a comfortable position**: Sit on the corner of one or more single-fold square blankets or lie down on your yoga mat with your knees bent. Rest your hands on your abdomen, one on top of the other or side by side, whichever feels most natural. Take several deep breaths, allowing yourself to settle. Focus on the contact between your hands and your body, imagining it as a bridge connecting your outer awareness to your inner consciousness.

- **Cultivate presence**: Breathe naturally through your nose and gently ask yourself, "Am I fully present in my body?" This question might feel unfamiliar or challenging at first, as we often lose touch with our physical sensations amidst the demands of daily life. With consistent practice, however, you'll develop a deeper awareness of the varying degrees of connection you have with your body, cultivating a stronger sense of presence over time.
- **Assess your energy level**: Do you feel full of energy, or are you completely drained? Observe your state without judgment or the need to analyze.
- **Notice the activity of your mind**: Are your thoughts racing, or does your mind feel sluggish? A restless mind often signals underlying anxiety. If a particular thought or concern occupies you, acknowledge it with kindness.
- **Check your nervous system**: Do you feel restlessness like a live wire or a buzzing sensation that's hard to calm? Or do you feel drained, as if your battery is empty and needs recharging?
- **Scan for physical tension or pain**: Direct your attention to areas of physical tension or discomfort. Identify any tightness or pain present in your body.
- **Relax your jaw**: Shift your attention to the outer muscles of your jaw, and consciously release any tension.
- **Focus on your abdomen**, home to your "second brain," the enteric nervous system. Is your belly tense or relaxed? Anxiety can increase stomach acidity, potentially disrupting the gut microbiome and leading to inflammation. Identifying and releasing this tension is a crucial step toward self-care.
- **Acknowledge your emotions**: What do you feel in this moment? Fear, anxiety, sadness, frustration? Simply recognize whatever arises with compassion.

When you've completed your check-in, gently roll onto your side. Take your time transitioning to a seated position, moving slowly and mindfully. Pause to notice any differences in how you feel compared to before the check-in.

In neuroscience, the Hawthorne effect suggests that directing attention inward can naturally facilitate changes from one moment to the next. Acknowledge these shifts: perhaps a sense of calm, groundedness, or increased presence. Practicing this mindful check-in before and after your Restorative Yoga sessions enables you to observe the practice's impact on your body, mind, and emotions.

Addressing Anxiety

Anxiety and fear are closely intertwined emotions, which is why our brain responds to them in similar ways. Fear is a primal response to a specific threat or dangerous situation, while anxiety arises from a perceived danger, even without an objective threat. Although anxiety can serve a physiological purpose by prompting adaptive behaviors after negative experiences, it becomes problematic when disproportionate to the perceived danger. As discussed in chapter 1, the brain's activation of the fight-or-flight response triggers a cascade of physiological reactions. The body scan practiced earlier is a powerful tool for developing self-awareness, known as interoception—the ability to perceive and assess our internal physiological state accurately.

When we experience anxiety, we often feel restless, struggle to focus, and find ourselves perpetually scanning the environment for potential threats. This hypervigilant state keeps us on edge, with racing thoughts fixated on future uncertainties and numerous "what if" scenarios. Anxiety can also cause irritability, physical tension, digestive discomfort due to increased gastric acid, and sleep disturbances, resulting in insomnia. To counteract these responses, it's essential to learn how to activate the parasympathetic nervous system in calm, low-stress situations, such as during a Restorative Yoga practice. With consistent practice, you can train yourself to access this calming response even in stressful moments, whether by observing your breath or taking a brief pause, such as resting your forehead on a desk.

This chapter introduces a sequence of poses designed to calm your mind, concluding with a variation of Savasana that opens the chest and supports deeper, easier breathing. This is to be complemented by a pranayama practice known as Visama Vritti (Unequal Breathing), a breathing technique that extends the exhale to twice the length of the inhale.

Practicing Visama Vritti (Unequal Breathing)

To practice Visama Vritti:

- Begin by gradually deepening your breath.
- Slowly lengthen your exhale until it becomes twice as long as your inhale.
- Alternate each deep breath with a normal breath to prevent self-competition and create space for slowing down and letting go.

Avoid forcing your breath, as this can lead to tension in the diaphragm, face, or neck, inadvertently stimulating the nervous system. Signs of discomfort might include difficulty breathing or feelings of anxiety about fully inhaling or exhaling. If this happens, return to your natural breathing rhythm and wait until you feel ready to try extending your exhale again.

Adho Mukha Swastikasana (Supported Forward Bend with Crossed Legs)

3–5 MINUTES

This gentle forward bend is a powerful pose for calming the mind, offering immediate relief during episodes of anxiety. The soothing pressure applied to the forehead activates the relaxation response, helping to ease mental tension. Additionally, this pose supports abdominal relaxation, making it effective for alleviating spasms or discomfort in the belly.

Compared to Upavistha Konasana, this variation is more accessible, as the knees remain comfortably bent, reducing strain in the hips and hamstrings while still allowing the spine to release forward with support.

CONTRAINDICATION

- spinal disc issues

PROPS NEEDED

1 yoga mat, 1 chair, 4–6 blankets, 1 eye pillow

SETTING UP THE POSE

- Place a chair at one end of your yoga mat and drape a single-fold square blanket over the seat for cushioning.
- Sit facing the chair on the corner of one or more single-fold square blankets to lift your pelvis. This elevation encourages a slight forward tilt, creating a gentle inward lumbar curve.
- Cross your legs at your ankles. If this feels uncomfortable, you can modify it by bringing one heel close to the perineum, with the sole of your foot gently resting against the inner thigh of the opposite leg. Place the other foot in front of the opposite ankle or shin, allowing both feet to rest comfortably without strain in Sukhasana (Easy Position, fig. 3.1).
- Fold a blanket lengthwise three times to create a narrow strip. Place the folded blanket horizontally across your abdomen, between your lower ribs and hip bones. Ensure it's under your abdomen, not under your hips. Take both ends of the blanket and wrap them around your pelvis, similar to tying a kimono belt. Secure it with a knot at your back, providing gentle compression to promote relaxation.
- Lean forward, folding your arms and sliding them under the folds of the blanket for added stability. Adjust your distance from the chair to find the most comfortable position while maintaining a lengthened lower back.

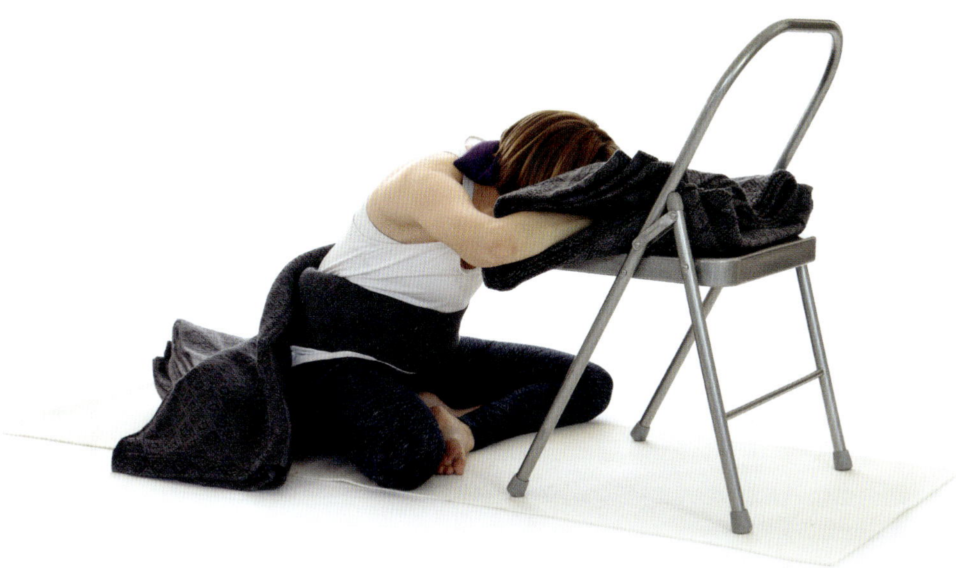

FIGURE 3.1 Audrey demonstrates Adho Mukha Swastikasana with the legs in Sukhasana, the forehead resting on a chair, and a rolled blanket around the belly to encourage deep relaxation.

- Rest your forehead on the blanket-covered seat of the chair. If this feels uncomfortable, turn your head to one side. Ensure your neck stays aligned and does not collapse; if it does, add an extra blanket on the chair for support.
- Cover yourself with a blanket for warmth and place an eye bag at the back of your neck for added comfort. Close your eyes, gently draw your chin slightly back and in, and settle into the pose.

GUIDING STUDENTS THROUGH RELAXATION

During the practice, you can use the following guidance to help students relax deeply and connect with the pose:

- Breathe naturally through your nose and let your attention drift to your forehead. Allow it to rest fully on the chair, immersing yourself in the physical sensations of the gentle pressure against the seat. Let this soothing contact quiet your mind and slow your thoughts.
- Feel the weight of the eye bag gently pressing against the back of your neck. Allow its soft presence to ease any tension, inviting your neck and shoulders to relax completely.
- Shift your awareness to the blanket wrapped around your abdomen. Sense the fabric's firm yet gentle support, encouraging your belly to soften and expand with each natural breath. Let the comforting embrace of the cotton belt create a sense of safety and ease.

- Bring your awareness to where your body meets the ground. Release all muscular effort in your thighs; they have no work to do here. Let your feet completely surrender, melting effortlessly into the earth.
- Midway through your practice, gently adjust your position by crossing your right ankle over your left, or vice versa, to restore balance. Once you've made this adjustment, return to stillness and settle even deeper into relaxation.

TRANSITIONING OUT OF THE POSE

- When it is time to come out of the pose, slowly bring your awareness back to the sensations of contact with the floor, the blankets, and the chair.
- Gently open your eyes.
- When you feel ready, press your hands into the chair to guide yourself back into a seated position with ease.

Salamba Bharadvajasana (Supported Reclining Twist)

3–5 MINUTES EACH SIDE

This gentle twist offers a wealth of benefits for both body and mind. By calming the nervous system and encouraging deeper, more effortless breathing, it helps restore balance and tranquility. The pose subtly massages the abdominal organs, supporting digestion and enhancing overall vitality.

Salamba Bharadvajasana also provides an opportunity to release deep-seated tension along the spine, heart, neck, and head. Through this release, the pose creates space for both physical and emotional openness. As we soften into the twist, we cultivate a profound sense of calm and receptivity, deepening our ability to listen—to ourselves and to those around us—with greater presence and compassion.

PROPS NEEDED

1 yoga mat, 2 bolsters, 3–5 blankets, 1 block if needed, 1 eye pillow

SETTING UP THE POSE

- Place one bolster widthwise at the top of your yoga mat. Position a second bolster lengthwise on top of the first, creating a 45-degree angle. If the second bolster sags in the middle under your weight, slide a yoga brick underneath for additional stability.
- Place a single-fold square blanket at the top of the second bolster, aligning one corner of the blanket with your sternum. This setup gently elevates your chest and head for greater comfort.
- To begin the twist to the right, sit on the floor with your legs extended to the left, at an angle greater than 90 degrees from the bolster to allow your spine to twist comfortably. Position your right hip against the short edge of the second bolster, ensuring there is no gap between your hip and the bolster. The greater trochanter—the outermost bony point of your hip—should be centered along the side of the bolster to provide even and stable support.
- Bend your knees so your right leg rests underneath your left, and point your feet toward the back of your mat.
- Place a single-fold rectangular blanket between your shins and feet for support. For additional hip opening, add another single-fold rectangular blanket between your shins.
- Turn your torso toward the bolster and place your fingertips on the floor on either side of it. Inhale deeply, pressing your hands into the ground to lift through the spine and create length. As you exhale, gently rotate

your torso from the pelvis, and begin to lower it onto the bolster. Bend your elbows and allow the body to soften into the support.

- It's important to initiate the twist from the pelvis, not from the upper body. Avoid anchoring your sitting bones while trying to twist from the shoulders, as this can create excessive tension in the sacroiliac (SI) joint. The sacroiliac joint is a joint of stability, not mobility. It allows for only a very small degree of movement—just enough to accommodate walking. Forcing a twist beyond this limited range can irritate or destabilize the joint, especially when the rotation is initiated from the thoracic spine instead of being guided by the natural motion of the pelvis.
- Rest your head in the same direction as your knees. For a deeper twist, you can turn your head in the opposite direction.
- Let your hands rest comfortably on the first bolster.
- Place an eye bag at the back of your neck and cover your lower back with a blanket to encourage deeper relaxation. Cover yourself completely to stay warm and comfortable throughout the pose.

GUIDING STUDENTS THROUGH RELAXATION

During the practice, you can use the following guidance to help students relax deeply and connect with the pose:

- Close your eyes and gently lower your chin toward your chest, signaling to your mind and body that you are transitioning from an outer-directed to an inner-directed awareness. This shift inward is key to restoring emotional balance.
- Begin by taking slow, deep breaths through your nose, allowing your body to settle fully into the twist. With each inhale, feel your rib cage expand outward and upward. With each exhale, let your ribs gently return toward your spine. Visualize your breath lengthening the sides of your body, helping to deepen the twist naturally.
- Bring your attention to the space between your shoulder blades. Imagine you could breathe through the back of your chest. With each inhale, visualize air entering gently through the back of the heart. With each exhale, let it flow forward, as if passing through the front of the heart and into the bolster.
- Let your breath dissolve any tension along your spine, behind your heart, and across your shoulders. Feel the gentle embrace of the bolster supporting your chest, encouraging your shoulders and arms to release fully, becoming free of any effort or work.

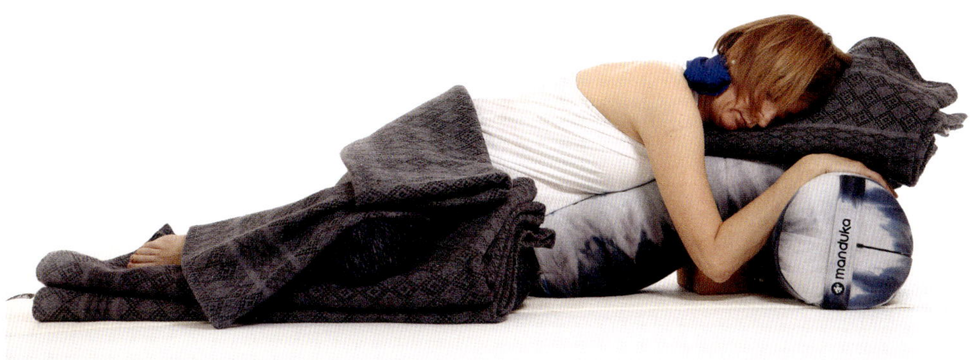

FIGURE 3.2 Audrey demonstrates Salamba Bharadvajasana on the left side with the torso resting at a 45-degree angle on a bolster, the head supported by folded blankets, and props under the legs for comfort.

- Visualize a gentle waterfall cascading over your ribs, flowing down toward the ground. With each breath, imagine this continual flow guiding you deeper into the twist, bringing a sense of ease and fluidity to your entire body.
- After three to five minutes, inhale deeply, place your palms on the floor under your shoulders, and press down to slowly sit up. Take your time to transition to the other side (fig. 3.2), and repeat the pose for another 3–5 minutes.

TRANSITIONING OUT OF THE POSE

- After completing the pose on both sides, reconnect with the space around you by taking slow, deep breaths.
- When you feel ready, place your palms on the floor under your shoulders.
- Inhale deeply and press down with your hands as you slowly sit up.

Ardha Viparita Karani (Half Legs Up the Wall Pose)

15–20 MINUTES

This pose is one of my favorite inversions because it's easy to practice without needing a wall. It helps you stay calm and relaxed throughout your session, allowing for smooth transitions to other poses without the need to stand up. This simplicity supports deep relaxation and makes your practice feel more seamless and restorative.

With the legs elevated above the heart and the heart above the head, this pose boosts blood circulation and encourages lymphatic drainage in the legs, abdomen, lungs, heart, and brain. It also has a soothing effect on the nervous system, leaving you feeling balanced, peaceful, and refreshed.

CONTRAINDICATIONS

- **pregnancy**: It's not recommended to practice inversions during pregnancy. (See "Avoiding Contraindications During Pregnancy" in chapter 4.)
- **menstruation**: Inversions are not recommended during menstruation, as they can disrupt the natural downward flow of energy. (See "During Menstruation" in chapter 4.)
- **sinusitis or cold**: The inverted position may exacerbate symptoms of sinus congestion.
- **gastroesophageal reflux disease (GERD)**: The inverted position can sometimes trigger or worsen acid reflux symptoms.
- **spinal conditions**: Individuals with spondylolysis or spondylolisthesis should consult a health care professional before practicing this pose.
- **eye conditions**: Those with retinal detachment or glaucoma should avoid inversions to prevent increased intraocular pressure.
- **hiatal hernia**: The position may place undue pressure on the abdomen, potentially aggravating this condition.

PROPS NEEDED

1 yoga mat, 1 chair, 1 bolster, 1 yoga belt, 6 blankets, 2 blocks, 1 sandbag

SETTING UP THE POSE

- Place a bolster lengthwise in the center of your mat in front of a chair. Cover the bolster with a single-fold rectangular blanket. (In fig. 3.3, the bolster is hidden under the blanket.)

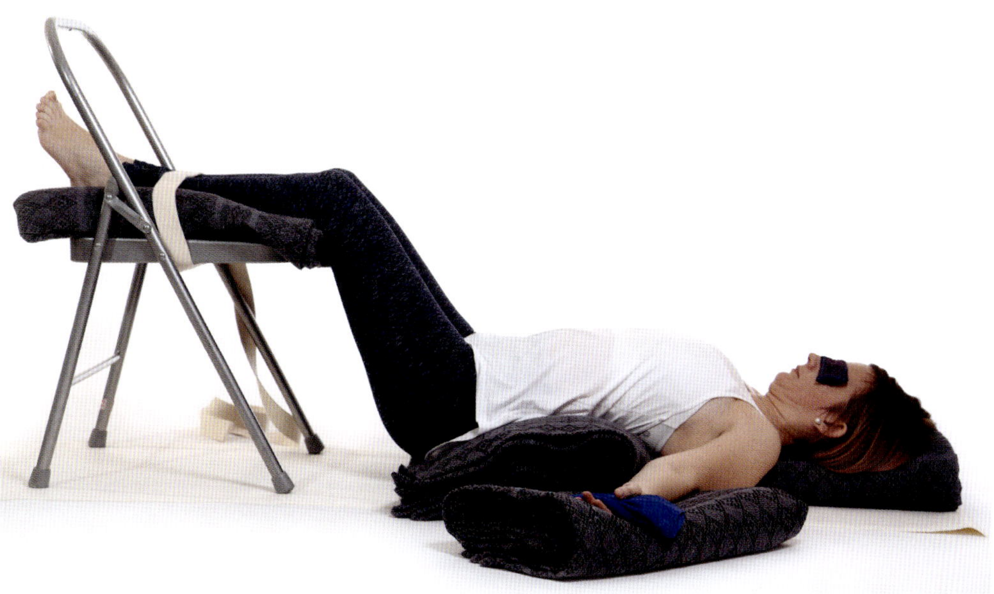

FIGURE 3.3 Audrey demonstrates Ardha Viparita Karani with the legs supported on a chair, a strap securing the calves, and the pelvis and lower ribs supported by a bolster and folded blanket to open the belly.

- Add a single-fold square blanket to the seat of the chair for cushioning. Loosely hook a yoga belt around the seat of the chair to keep your legs in position during the pose.
- Place a double-fold blanket perpendicular to the bolster, just in front of it, to support your shoulders and head.
- Sit on the bolster and place your lower legs on the chair seat. Ensure the backs of your knees are fully supported by the chair seat and that your heels are aligned horizontally with your knees. The heels should rest on the blanket, not dangle in the air.
- Gently turn your shins inward and secure a yoga belt around your legs just below the knees to support alignment and stability. This subtle internal rotation of the thighs encourages a gentle backbend through the lumbar spine, helping the front body to open with ease.
- Position your thighs at a 45-degree angle to the floor for optimal relaxation. Avoid positioning your thighs at a 90-degree angle to prevent strain on your lower back and legs.
- Make sure your pelvis and lower ribs are supported by the bolster, while your shoulders and head rest on the blanket. Your pubic bone should be at the same level as your navel or slightly lower.

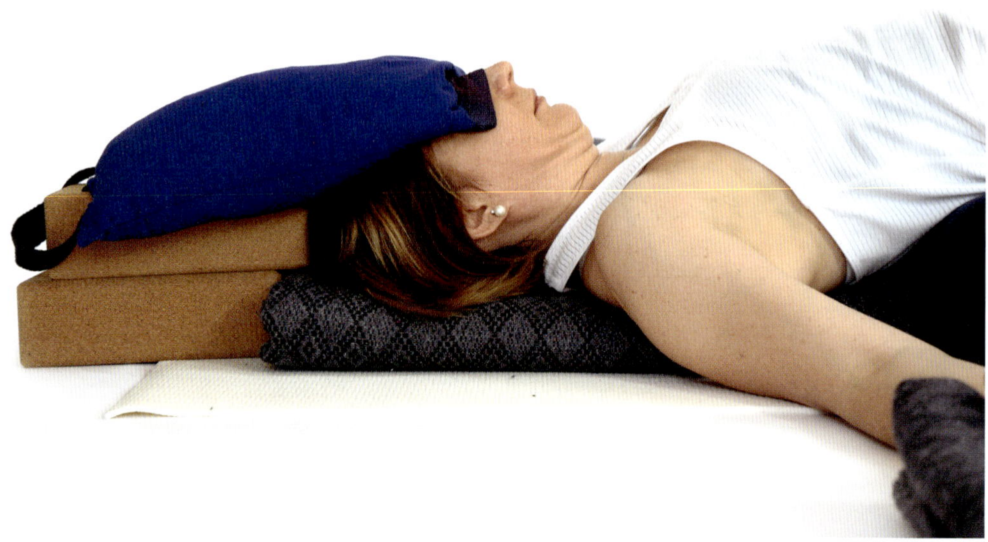

FIGURE 3.4 Audrey demonstrates a head-support setup in Ardha Viparita Karani using two cork bricks and a weighted sandbag over the forehead to provide grounding.

- Rest your arms at your sides and use two double-fold blankets to support them (fig. 3.3).
- Place two yoga bricks above your head, ensuring they do not touch it. Place a sandbag on top of the bricks, with one-third of the weight gently resting on your forehead to calm your mind (fig. 3.4).
- Check that your body is symmetrical, cover yourself with a blanket, and place an eye pillow over your eyes.

GUIDING STUDENTS THROUGH RELAXATION

During the practice, you can use the following guidance to help students relax deeply and connect with the pose:

- Begin by bringing your awareness to the back of your body. Slowly scan from heels to head, noticing all the places where your body connects with the props.
- Focus on your heels. As you exhale, feel them dropping into the chair, releasing any tension. Notice how the backs of your legs are gently held by the chair and strap. Let your shins relax into the belt, allowing your legs to completely rest.
- Shift your attention to your pelvis resting on the bolster. With each inhale, soften your belly; with each exhale, feel it settle gently into your pelvis and hips. Sense the bolster supporting your lower ribs,

and observe how your upper back rests comfortably against the blanket.

- As your upper back broadens, feel your neck relax and your throat open, allowing the nape and back of your head to be gently cradled by the blanket. Trust the ground to hold you completely, letting your breath flow naturally in and out.
- Turn your focus to your breath. Notice where it naturally expands in your back. With each inhale, feel your back widen and your ribs gently open. With each exhale, soften further into the support of the props and the ground.
- As you rest here, bring awareness to the connection of your breath, your body, and the ground. Feel your back widen with each breath, softening into the support.

TRANSITIONING OUT OF THE POSE

- When it is time to come out of the pose, bring your awareness back to the sensations of contact with the floor and the props.
- Slowly remove the eye bag and the sandbag and allow your eyes to open softly, adjusting gradually to the light.
- Gently slip your legs out from the belt.
- Very slowly, slide yourself backward toward your head until your entire back is resting on the floor.
- Bend your knees and remain in this position for a few moments.
- When you feel ready, roll onto your side and return to a seated position, using your hands for support.

Savasana for Pranayama (Corpse Pose with Breathing)

20–25 MINUTES

This variation promotes deeper, more expansive breathing and is especially beneficial for practitioners who may struggle to stay awake during traditional Savasana. This variation provides gentle support to the upper body, encouraging alert relaxation while maintaining a sense of ease and comfort.

CONTRAINDICATION

After the second trimester of pregnancy, it is recommended to practice Side-Lying Savasana on your left side (fig. 4.20).

PROPS NEEDED

1 yoga mat, 1 bolster, 5 blankets, 3 eye pillows

SETTING UP THE POSE

- Arrange three single-fold rectangular blankets in a stepped formation on your mat with the thin edges toward your body and the thick edges toward your head. Leave a space of 4–6 inches between each blanket. Turn the top edge of the uppermost blanket under to create a gentle incline for supporting the head.
- Sit on the mat (not on the blankets) with your pelvis touching the bottom edge of the lowest blanket. Lie back onto the blankets, ensuring your body aligns with the midline of the setup. Adjust as needed so the lowest blanket supports your pelvis, the second supports your lower back, and the third supports your upper back and head.
- Arrange the top edge of the uppermost blanket to comfortably support your head and neck, extending the blanket down to the tops of your shoulders. Ensure your chin is slightly lower than your forehead to maintain optimal alignment.
- Place a bolster under the backs of your knees to reduce tension in the lower back. Position a rolled blanket under your Achilles tendons so your heels are gently suspended above the mat.
- Move your arms away from your torso to ensure unrestricted rib movement as you breathe. For added comfort, rest your hands on two folded eye pillows (fig. 3.5).
- Cover yourself with a blanket to stay warm. Close your eyes, and place an eye bag over them to deepen your relaxation.

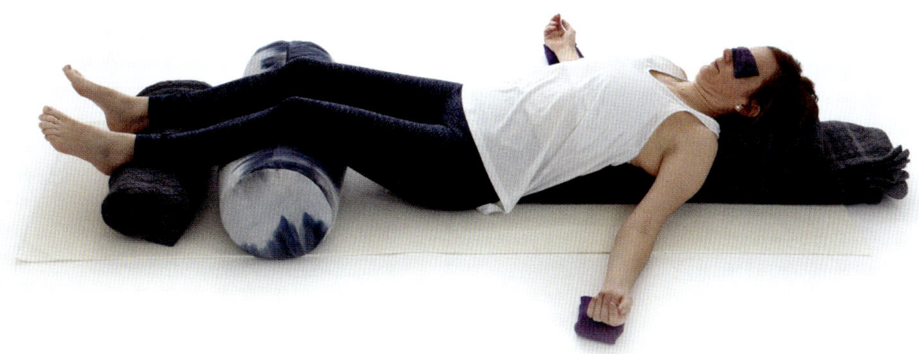

FIGURE 3.5 Audrey demonstrates Savasana for Pranayama with the chest elevated by three folded blankets stacked in a stair-step shape to gently open the front body.

GUIDING STUDENTS THROUGH RELAXATION

During the practice, you can use the following guidance to help students relax deeply and connect with the pose:

- Start by bringing your attention to the overall condition of your body. Allow any muscular tension to dissolve naturally. Adjust your position if needed to ensure you are completely at ease and free of resistance. Once a sense of calm has settled, gently shift your focus to your breathing. At this stage, it's important not to alter the natural rhythm of your breath. Simply allow it to flow naturally.
- Observe the sensations of your breath. Follow its journey as it moves from your nostrils to your lungs, and from your lungs back to your nostrils. Notice the subtle difference in temperature between the inhale and exhale. Feel the quiet movements in your body: the gentle dilation of your nostrils, the expansion of your rib cage, the lift of your ribs, and the rise and fall of your abdomen.
- Watch your breath as if you were a detached observer, simply noticing its natural flow for a few moments without judgment or control.
- Next, begin to count the length of your inhale and exhale. Gradually extend both, increasing each by a couple of counts. Let this extension unfold effortlessly.
- As you inhale, feel your ribs expanding outward and upward as air fills your lungs. Allow this movement to happen naturally. Keep your abdomen passive.
- As you exhale, relax all the muscles in your chest. Notice your rib cage gently contracting as the air flows out of your lungs.
- Take a normal breath in and out before starting the next cycle.

- Repeat this pattern, gradually allowing your chest to expand more with each inhale. Exhale slowly until a natural breath takes over.
- Once your breath is longer but still stable, begin extending the exhale by one count. For instance, if you inhale for two counts, exhale for three. If you inhale for three counts, exhale for four; and so on. Between each deep breath, allow a normal breath to ensure ease and comfort.
- If your breathing remains comfortable, transition to an even longer exhale, making it two counts longer than your inhale. Stay within your comfort range. Signs of discomfort might include difficult breathing or anxiety about being able to breathe in again or exhale fully. If you experience any discomfort, return to the last breath ratio that felt good to you.
- If you still feel at ease, gradually lengthen your exhale until it becomes twice as long as your inhale. For instance, if you inhale for two counts, exhale for four; if you inhale for three counts, exhale for six, and so on. Take a normal breath between each cycle to remain at ease.
- Continue this pattern for 3–5 minutes. When you feel ready, let your breath return to its natural rhythm. Remain in this pose for an additional 15–20 minutes, allowing your body and mind to integrate the calming effects of the practice.

TRANSITIONING OUT OF THE POSE

- As your practice comes to an end, bring your awareness back to the sensations of contact with the floor and the props. Observe your breath: its quality, its shape, its texture.
- Turn your knees inward and bring your lower back onto the blankets.
- Bend one knee, then the other, and place your feet on the bolster.
- Roll onto the side of your choice, letting your eye bag fall gently to the ground.
- When you feel ready, slowly return to a seated position, pressing the hand closest to your chest into the floor for support while using the other hand to help you sit up.
- With your eyes still closed, take a few moments to check-in, noticing any changes that may have occurred.

If you fall asleep during one of the poses, remember that it's perfectly fine—especially if you've been struggling with sleep for months or are going through particularly challenging times. In such moments, this practice can offer an opportunity for deep rest.

That said, the primary aim of this practice is to help you release long-held tensions, and achieving this requires staying consciously present throughout the process. It's important to recognize that relaxation and sleep are two distinct physiological needs, much like eating and drinking. One cannot substitute for the other.

If You Suffer from Insomnia

Improving your sleep takes patience and consistency. Here are some practical tips to help you sleep better and gradually increase your hours of rest, with the ultimate goal of achieving the eight consecutive hours recommended by sleep specialists:

- **Maintain a consistent bedtime:** Go to bed at the same time every night to establish a regular sleep schedule.
- **Wake up at the same time every morning:** Keep your wake-up time consistent, including on weekends, to regulate your internal clock.
- **Create an eight-hour sleep window:** Ensure you allocate enough time for 8 hours of uninterrupted sleep, minimizing nighttime awakenings.
- **Avoid naps:** If you feel tired during the day, opt for a brief Restorative Yoga session with a timer instead of napping.
- **Limit stimulants:** Steer clear of caffeine, alcohol, dark chocolate, and nicotine, especially in the afternoon and evening.
- **Take vitamin D in the morning:** This timing helps avoid interference with melatonin production, the hormone essential for regulating sleep.
- **Expose yourself to natural daylight:** Spend at least 30 minutes in the morning sunlight to support the natural release of melatonin in the evening.
- **Finish eating well before bedtime:** Have your last meal 2–3 hours before sleeping to prevent digestion from interfering with restful sleep.
- **Avoid intense exercise before bed:** Refrain from engaging in physical activity within 2 hours of bedtime.
- **Limit exposure to blue light:** Reduce screen time from phones, computers, tablets, or TVs at least 2 hours before bed as blue light suppresses melatonin production.
- **Use blue light–blocking glasses:** If avoiding screens isn't possible, use blue light–blocking glasses to mitigate the effects.
- **Dim the lights in the evening:** Lower the lighting in your home 90 minutes before bed to signal to your body that it's time to wind down.

- **Optimize your bedroom temperature:** Keep the room cool, ideally 64–68°F, to prevent heat from raising cortisol levels and disrupting sleep.
- **Develop a bedtime relaxation routine:** Practice a calming Restorative Yoga pose before sleeping to release physical tension and prepare your body and mind for rest.
- **Sleep on your side:** Use a body pillow or a maternity pillow to support your body and enhance comfort.
- **Practice Bhramari breathing:** This soothing breath technique can help quiet your mind and relax your body. Use it before bed or during nighttime awakenings to ease yourself back into sleep.

Bhramari Pranayama (Bee's Breath)

The word *bhramari*, in Sanskrit, means "bee's breath." As described by Swami Sivananda, "The inhale is quick and forceful.... The exhale, very slow, resembles the humming of the female bee."[1] Practicing Bhramari for just a few minutes can create a profound calming effect on the mind, fostering a deep sense of tranquility and well-being. It is particularly effective for alleviating insomnia and promoting restful sleep.

THE SCIENCE BEHIND BHRAMARI

The gentle humming sound produced during Bhramari breathing stimulates the vagus nerve, a crucial component of the parasympathetic nervous system, responsible for the body's rest-and-digest response. The vibrations from humming help activate this nerve, promoting relaxation, reducing stress, and restoring balance to the nervous system.[2]

Additionally, Bhramari Pranayama significantly enhances the production of nitric oxide in the nasal passages—up to fifteen times more than during normal breathing.[3] Nitric oxide is an important signaling molecule with multiple benefits, including:

- **vasodilation**: It widens blood vessels, improving circulation.
- **anti-inflammatory effects**: It helps reduce inflammation in the body.
- **enhanced oxygen uptake**: It supports overall cardiovascular health.

For those who struggle with insomnia, practicing Bhramari breathing before bedtime can be particularly beneficial.

HOW TO PRACTICE BHRAMARI BREATHING

1. Prepare

- Lie down comfortably in Savasana for Pranayama.
- Begin by breathing naturally, observing the flow of your breath without attempting to change it. Allow a sense of calm to envelop your body and mind.

2. Start the Breath Cycle

- Take a normal deep breath in through your nose.
- As you exhale slowly, produce a humming sound from the back of your throat, similar to the internalized sound of the mantra "Om." The tone should fall between "ah" and "oh," and your soft palate should remain relaxed, similar to the sensation of yawning with a closed mouth.

3. Repeat

- Complete this cycle at least six times, or as many as feels comfortable.

4. Relax

- After completing the cycles, remain in Savasana for 15–20 minutes, allowing your breath to return to its natural rhythm and your body to integrate the calming effects.

Tips for Nighttime Awakenings

If you awaken during the night, you can practice Bhramari breathing while lying in bed. The soothing vibrations and deep exhalations can help ease your mind and guide you back into restful sleep. By incorporating Bhramari Pranayama into your routine, you not only support better sleep but also nurture your overall mental and physical well-being.

Restorative Yoga Sequences for Managing Anxiety

The following are additional sequences to help calm anxiety and manage insomnia. Some are shorter, recognizing that it can be challenging to remain still for twenty minutes when feeling anxious. Gradually, and at your own pace, you will be able to extend the duration of your practice.

SEQUENCE 2: 25–30 MINUTES

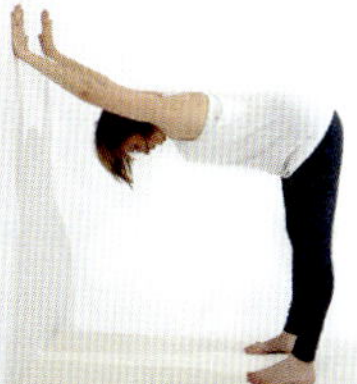

Ardha Svanasana (page 158)
2–3 minutes

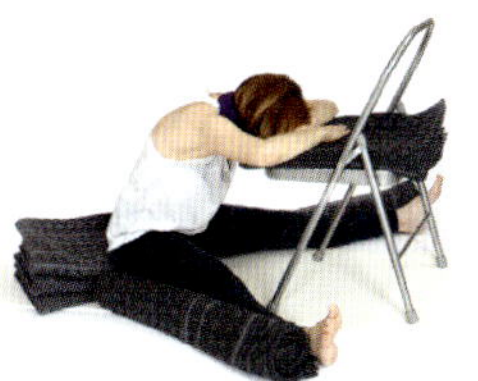

Salamba Upavistha Konasana (page 38)
2–5 minutes

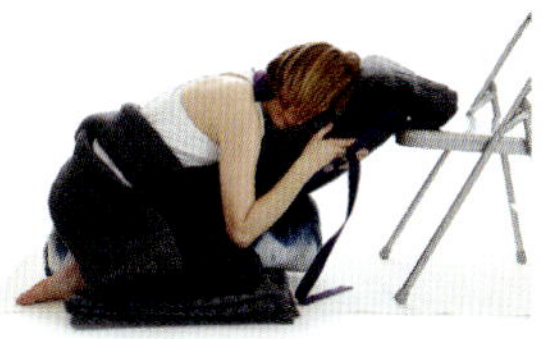

Salamba Balasana with Two Bolsters (page 116)
5 minutes each side

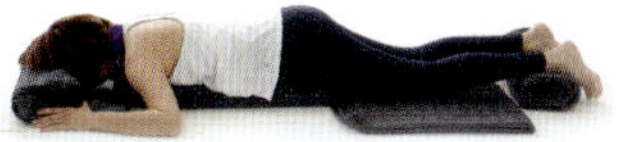

Adho Mukha Savasana with One Bolster (page 150)
10–15 minutes

SEQUENCE 3: 35–45 MINUTES

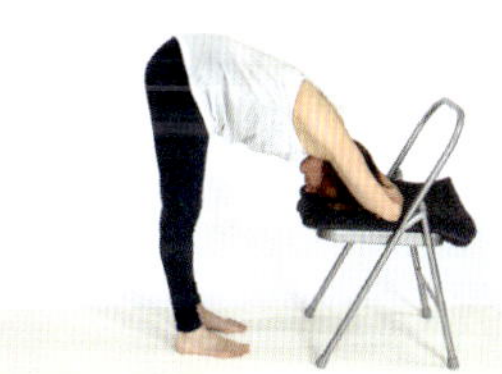

Salamba Uttanasana (page 71)
2–3 minutes

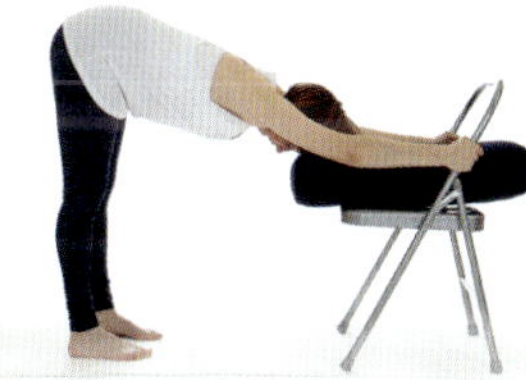

Salamba Adho Mukha Svanasana (page 180)
2–3 minutes

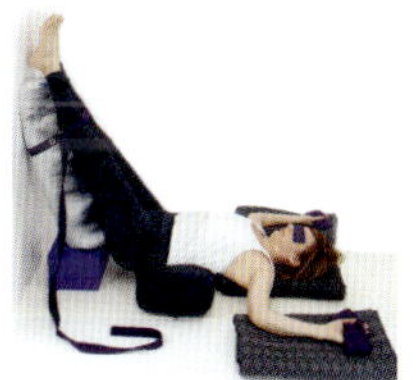

Viparita Karani (page 183)
10–15 minutes

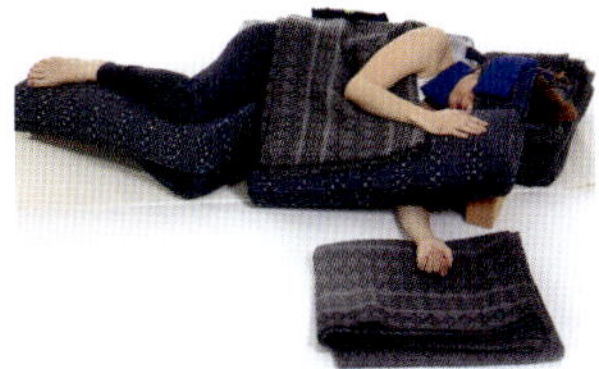

Side-Lying Savasana (page 168)
20–25 minutes

SEQUENCE 4: 40–50 MINUTES

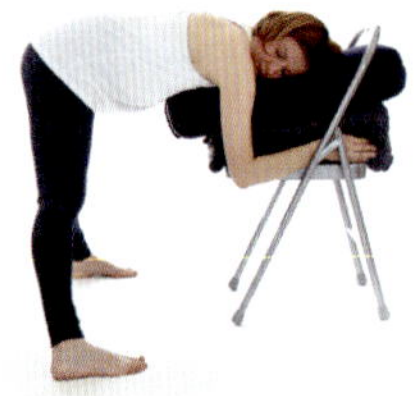

Salamba Prasarita Padottanasana with a Chair (page 177) 2–3 minutes

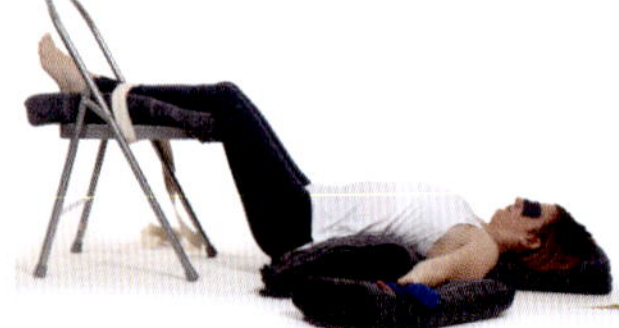

Ardha Viparita Karani (page 56)
8–15 minutes

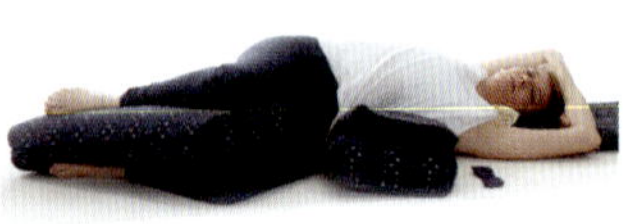

Salamba Jathara Parivartanasana (page 35)
3 minutes each side

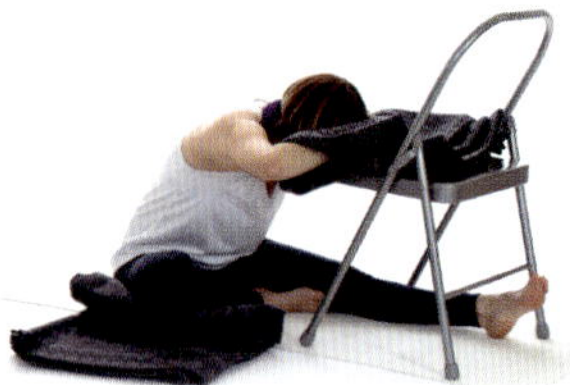

Salamba Janu Sirsasana (page 74)
2–3 minutes each side

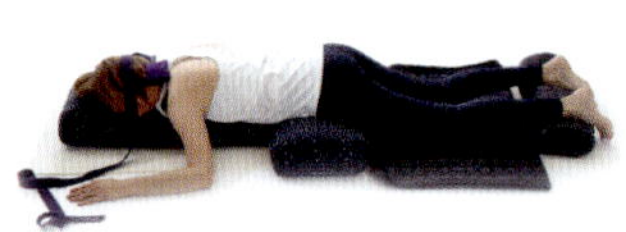

Adho Mukha Savasana with Two Bolsters (page 149)
20 minutes

SEQUENCE 5 FOR ADVANCED STUDENTS

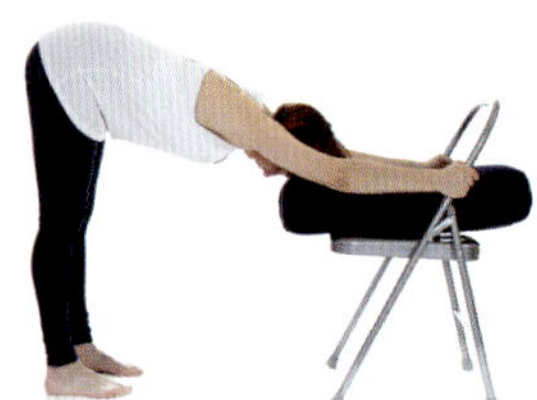

Salamba Adho Mukha Svanasana (page 180)
2–3 minutes

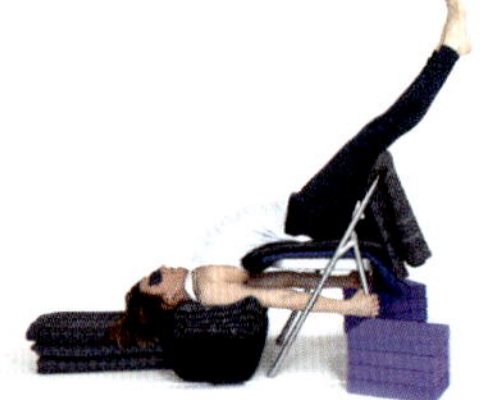

Salamba Sarvangasana (page 129)
2–15 minutes

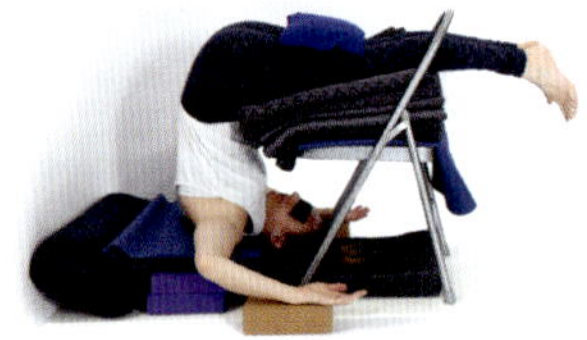

Ardha Halasana (page 141)
10–15 minutes

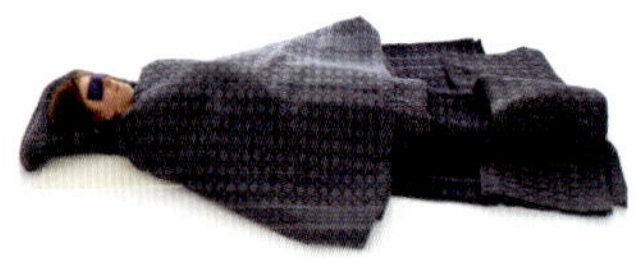

Swaddled Savasana (page 100)
20–25 minutes

Addressing Anger

Our daily lives are full of moments that create emotional tension, making it easy to feel off balance and frustrated. A delayed project or a disagreement can quickly trigger anger, leading to a defensive reaction. Physically our heart rate speeds up, tension builds, and we may feel a rush of heat. Mentally we focus on others' actions, judging them harshly and replaying past frustrations.

At its core, anger is a natural emotion that arises when our needs are unmet. However, when anger takes hold it often diverts us from finding constructive solutions. Instead our thoughts become trapped in cycles of blame, judgment, and frustration. We may dwell on beliefs like "They shouldn't have acted that way," which pulls us further away from understanding our own authentic needs.

Breaking free from this cycle requires a conscious pause, a moment to reconnect with what we truly need. For many of us, this process is challenging because we've been conditioned to suppress our own needs, prioritizing others' demands instead. Recognizing and honoring these needs is a powerful step toward emotional balance. These needs may include:

- **autonomy**: Pursuing our dreams, goals, and values.
- **celebration**: Acknowledging achievements or processing loss.
- **integrity**: Cultivating authenticity, creativity, meaning, and self-esteem.
- **interdependence**: Experiencing closeness, emotional safety, honesty, love, and respect.
- **physical nourishment**: Receiving air, food, movement, exercise, and protection.
- **play and spiritual connection**: Finding beauty, harmony, inspiration, order, and peace.

When we connect with these underlying needs, anger often transforms into other emotions, such as sadness, fear, or pain, feelings that motivate us to act in ways that genuinely address our needs. While anger tends to drive us toward blame and punishment, reconnecting with our emotions allows us to approach situations with empathy and clarity.

As Judith Hanson Lasater, a student of Marshall B. Rosenberg, the creator of Nonviolent Communication, explains in her book *What We Say Matters*, empathy is the key to moving beyond irritation.[4] Cultivating empathy for ourselves and others helps us shift our reactions, creating space for compassion and understanding.

The Restorative Yoga sequence in this chapter is designed to ground you, process emotional experiences, and foster self-compassion. By stimulating the parasympathetic nervous system, the body's rest-and-digest response, this practice allows you to:

- gain clarity about behavioral patterns
- reduce defensiveness
- lessen judgmental thinking
- cultivate deeper compassion
- approach challenges with creativity and calm

Through this practice, you can gradually transform your interactions, even with those who trigger deeply ingrained reactions. By grounding yourself in presence and empathy, you create a foundation for more conscious and compassionate connections.

Salamba Uttanasana (Supported Standing Forward Bend)

2–3 MINUTES

This forward fold offers a deeply calming effect on the mind, making it especially effective for silencing the inner critic and fostering mental clarity. Physically, Uttanasana helps release tension in the back, alleviates stomach discomfort, and provides a sense of grounding, anchoring you firmly in the present moment.

CONTRAINDICATIONS

- herniated disc
- sacroiliac dysfunction
- radiating pain in the arms or legs

For those experiencing back pain, limited mobility in forward bends, or tight hamstrings, consider practicing Ardha Svanasana instead (fig. 4.17). This alternative pose offers similar benefits while maintaining comfort and safety.

PROPS NEEDED

1 yoga mat, 1 chair, 1–2 blankets

SETTING UP THE POSE

- Place a sturdy chair on a nonslip yoga mat with the seat facing you. For added comfort, cover the chair seat with a single-fold square blanket.
- Stand facing the chair with your feet hip width apart, 14–18 inches. Ensure the outer edges of your feet are parallel to the edges of the mat to facilitate the movement of your pelvis around the heads of the femurs.
- Inhale deeply and extend your arms upward over your head. Gently hold your elbows with opposite hands, creating a soft stretch through the sides of your body (fig. 3.6).
- As you exhale, bend forward from your hip joints, keep your chin slightly down, and maintain the natural curves in your spine. Allow the natural weight of your upper body to guide you into the pose. Keep your head and neck relaxed as you move into the fold.
- Rest the top of your forehead, at the hairline, on the chair seat. Place your folded arms on the chair seat in front of you, letting them rest comfortably. Adjust your position to ensure your neck is in flexion. If your neck is in extension, gently draw your chin toward your heart for proper alignment. Close your eyes and take slow, deep breaths. Allow your body to soften as you settle into the pose (fig. 3.7).

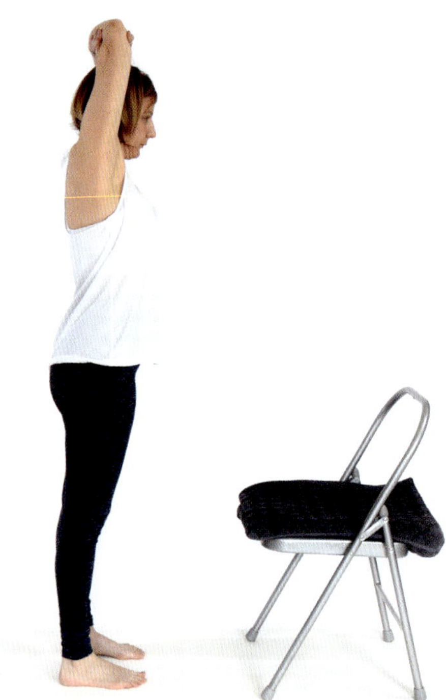

FIGURE 3.6 Audrey demonstrates a standing preparatory movement for Salamba Uttanasana in front of a chair covered with a folded blanket.

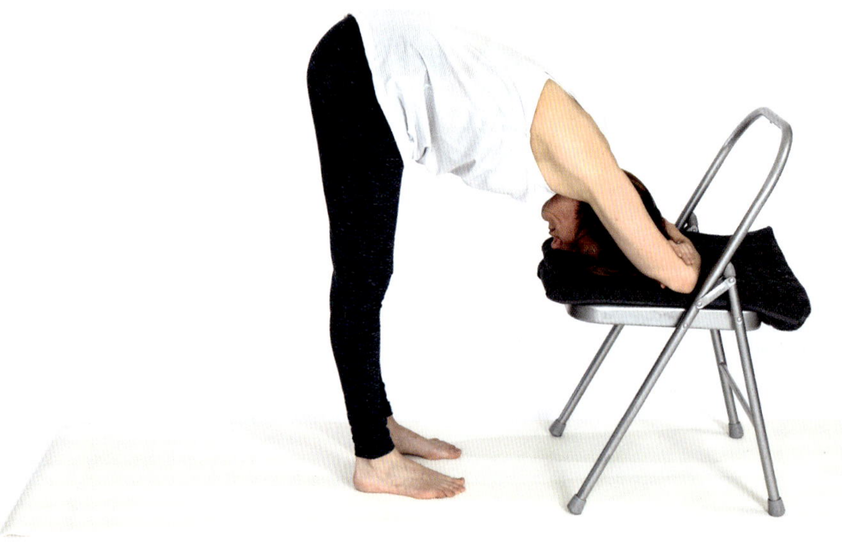

FIGURE 3.7 Audrey demonstrates Salamba Uttanasana with the forehead resting on a folded blanket on a chair, with a straight line in the ankles, knees, and hips, and a soft curve in the back to encourage introversion.

GUIDING STUDENTS THROUGH RELAXATION

During the practice, you can use the following guidance to help students relax deeply and connect with the pose:

- Breathe naturally through your nose and gently bring your attention to your head. Allow it to rest completely on the chair. With each exhale, release any tension in your face, neck, and shoulders. Let your forearms soften, and surrender fully onto the seat of the chair.
- Shift your awareness to your back, and direct your breath into this area. With every exhale, feel tension melting away, leaving your back soft, open, and at ease.
- Bring your attention to your connection with the ground. Imagine roots growing from the soles of your feet, reaching deep into the earth and anchoring you.
- Take a few quiet moments to savor this sensation of grounding, stability, and connection. Feel the earth offering steady and reliable support.

TRANSITIONING OUT OF THE POSE

- Gently open your eyes and take a moment to reconnect with the space around you.
- When you feel ready, place your hands on the sides of the chair seat and straighten your arms, creating a sense of stability.
- On your next inhale, lengthen the front of your torso, allowing your spine to return to its natural neutral curve.
- Gradually lift your upper body, maintaining this length, and come up to a standing position with ease and control.
- Take a few breaths to settle before transitioning into the next pose.

Salamba Janu Sirsasana (Supported Head-to-Knee Pose)

3–4 MINUTES EACH SIDE

This pose offers a gentle yet effective stretch for the lower-back muscles, enhancing hip joint flexibility and soothing the abdominal organs. This pose is particularly beneficial for calming the mind, lowering blood pressure, and fostering a deep sense of inward-focused awareness. Additionally, it stimulates the liver, spleen, and kidneys, supporting overall vitality and internal balance.

CONTRAINDICATIONS

- herniated disc
- lower-back pain
- tight hamstrings or hips
- knee injuries or pain

PROPS NEEDED

1 yoga mat, 1 chair, 3 blankets, 1 eye pillow

SETTING UP THE POSE

- Place a chair at one end of your yoga mat with the seat facing you. For added comfort, cover the chair seat with a single-fold square blanket.
- Sit on the floor with your legs extended under the chair and your torso upright.
- Inhale, and with an exhale, bend your right knee slightly. Use the middle and third fingers of your right hand to feel behind your right knee. Locate the ligaments on the back of the left side of the knee and gently pull them outward to encourage the shin to rotate naturally outward and downward.
- Bring your right foot toward your groin, angling it slightly diagonally. If your right knee does not touch the floor, place a rolled blanket underneath it for support.
- Sit just in front of your sitting bones to maintain proper pelvic alignment.
- Place your palms on the floor beside your hips with your fingers pointing forward.
- Inhale deeply, and as you exhale, press your hands into the floor to stretch upward through the sides and back of your body.
- Lengthen the front of your torso, lifting from the pubic bone upward to create space in your spine.

- Anchor firmly through the root of your right hip joint. Allow the right pelvis to lift slightly and roll over the stationary right femur to avoid straining the sacroiliac joint.
- Inhale deeply, and as you exhale, gently rotate your torso to the left from the pelvis. Take the right side of your pelvis with you during this slight twist.
- Slowly begin to fold forward, ensuring the movement originates from your right pelvis and hip joint.
- Align your breastbone with the inside of your extended left thigh.
- Rest your forehead on the chair seat and place your arms on the chair in front of your head. Tuck your hands under the blanket on the seat to keep them secure.
- Adjust the distance between your body and the chair as needed to ensure comfort and an elongated lower back (fig. 3.8).
- Ensure your neck remains long and does not collapse while your forehead rests on the chair. If necessary, add an additional blanket to the chair seat to bring the support closer to your head.
- Cover yourself with a blanket to stay warm. Place an eye pillow at the back of your neck to encourage deeper relaxation. Close your eyes, allowing the props and pose to fully support you. Adjust your position or props if any part of your body feels tense or unsupported.

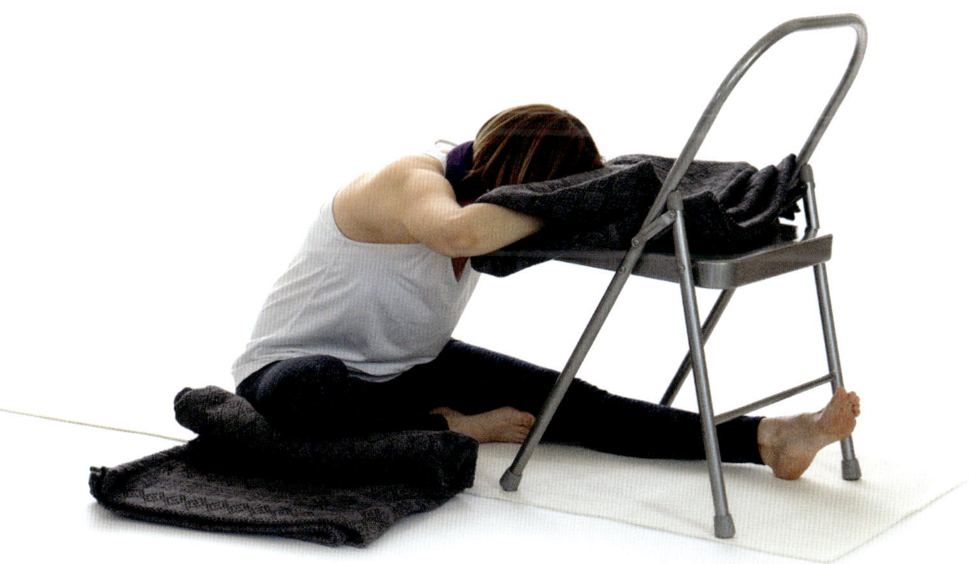

FIGURE 3.8 Audrey demonstrates Salamba Janu Sirsasana with the forehead resting on a chair and a soft curve in the back to support introspection and moderation.

GUIDING STUDENTS THROUGH RELAXATION

During the practice, you can use the following guidance to help students relax deeply and connect with the pose:

- Begin by taking several deep, slow breaths through your nose, allowing each exhale to guide your body and mind into relaxation. Feel the steady rhythm of your breath creating space within you.
- Recognize that anger often manifests as tension in the body, particularly in the shoulders. With your next exhale, consciously soften your shoulder muscles, letting go of any tightness or rigidity. Imagine a warm wave of relaxation melting away tension with every breath.
- Bring your awareness to your back and spine. Allow the muscles along your spine to gently release, letting your back round naturally and open. With each inhale, invite a sense of ease to flow through your entire back, and with each exhale, surrender more deeply into the pose.
- Shift your attention to your hips and legs. Feel the earth supporting your sitting bones, legs, and feet. Your muscles do not need to work—allow them to fully relax.
- Let your jaw, forehead, and throat soften. Notice if you're holding subtle tension in these areas, and with each breath, release them. Allow your face to relax completely, creating a sense of inner calm.
- As you settle into the pose, bring awareness to your breath. Feel it moving through your back, ribs, and chest, gently expanding and releasing. Observe the quiet rhythm of your inhales and exhales, allowing you to sink deeper into stillness.
- Stay here for several minutes, breathing deeply and allowing the pose to nourish your body and mind. Each breath offers an opportunity to soften, release, and let go.
- When you feel ready to come out of the pose, take a deep inhale and gently lift yourself back up, using your hands for support. Move slowly and with care.
- Switch to the left side and repeat the pose for balance and symmetry.

TRANSITIONING OUT OF THE POSE

- After completing the pose on both sides, take a moment to reconnect with the space around you by taking slow, deep breaths.
- When you feel ready, inhale deeply, exhale fully, and gently lift yourself back up, using your hands for support.
- Extend your left leg, returning to an upright seated position. Pause here for a few moments to let your body adjust and absorb the effects of the pose before moving to your next pose.

Salamba Navasana (Supported Boat Pose) with Bent Legs

20–25 MINUTES

This supported variation of Navasana emphasizes relaxation and grounding rather than the core engagement typically associated with the traditional Navasana. The unique position of the body and the angle of the legs work together to release tension in the psoas muscles, a crucial muscle group that connects the upper to the lower halves of the body. These muscles influence how we move, how we breathe, and even how we feel.

UNDERSTANDING THE PSOAS MUSCLES

To appreciate the importance of the psoas, it helps to understand their anatomy and function. On each side of the body, there are two psoas muscles:

- **psoas major**: A large, powerful muscle that begins in the lower spine, runs through the pelvis, and attaches to the top of the thigh bone (the femur).
- **psoas minor**: A smaller muscle, present in some but not all people, located in front of the psoas major.

Together, these muscles extend along the back of the lower spine (the lumbar curve) and play a key role in stabilizing the body. The psoas major merges with the iliacus muscle beneath the inguinal ligament to form the iliopsoas, which is crucial for hip flexion and smooth movement.

What Do the Psoas Muscles Do?

The psoas muscles are remarkable in their role supporting both physical movement and instinctive responses.

- **facilitate movement**: They are the primary muscles for lifting the leg, bending the hip, and stabilizing the spine.
- **respond to stress**: Connected to the nervous system, the psoas plays a key role in the body's fight-flight-freeze response. When we sense danger, the psoas may contract to prepare for action like running or for immobilization like curling into a protective pose.
- **influence breathing**: Because of their proximity to the diaphragm, tight psoas muscles can restrict deep breathing, making it harder to relax fully.

THE IMPACT OF MODERN HABITS

In today's lifestyle, habits like sitting for long hours, driving, or walking on hard surfaces often keep the psoas in a state of chronic tension.[5] Over time, this can lead to:

- lower-back pain

- physical discomfort and stiffness
- digestion issues, as the psoas muscles are part of the abdominal wall
- difficulty breathing deeply

THE BENEFITS OF RELAXING THE PSOAS

Persistent tension in the psoas signals to the body that it is in a constant state of alert. However, releasing and softening these muscles through restorative practices like Salamba Navasana creates a profound sense of safety and stability.

This release fosters deeper breathing, a greater sense of presence, and a feeling of being grounded. In this way, the practice not only alleviates physical discomfort but also nurtures emotional balance, encouraging more harmonious interactions with ourselves and others in daily life.

PROPS NEEDED

1 yoga mat, 2 bolsters, 6 blocks, 3 bricks, 4–5 blankets, 3 eye bags

SETTING UP THE POSE

- Start by placing two blocks lengthwise on your yoga mat, stacked one on top of the other. Add a brick horizontally on top of the blocks. Then position a bolster lengthwise on top of the brick to create a 45-degree angle (fig. 3.9). Alternatively, you can use a chair and a bolster to achieve the same angle (fig. 3.10).
- Cover the bolster and the floor with a blanket folded in half widthwise to provide extra comfort for your back.

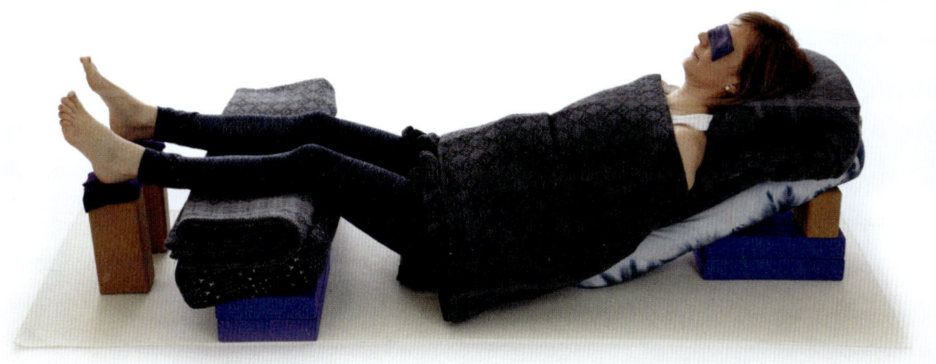

FIGURE 3.9 Audrey demonstrates Salamba Navasana with the torso supported at a 45-degree angle, the legs bent and supported to relax the psoas, and a wrap blanket around the arms for warmth and containment.

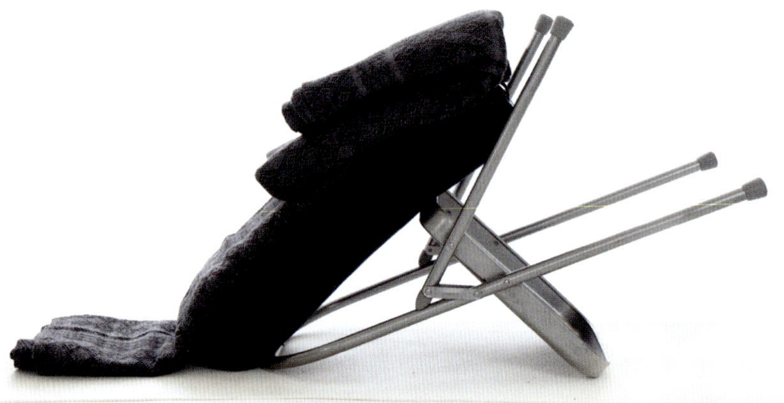

FIGURE 3.10 Setup for Salamba Navasana with the chair tilted back at a 45-degree angle, a bolster and folded blankets to support the spine, and padding under the chair for comfort.

- At the top of the bolster, add a standard-fold blanket folded into two layers. The higher layer should support your head with the thick edge placed under the C7 vertebra for optimal support, while the lower layer supports the top of your shoulder blades with its thin edge.
- Arrange four blocks to support another bolster and a single-fold rectangular blanket. Place two vertical bricks at the end of the bolster and top them with two folded eye pillows to support your heels.
- Sit in front of the first bolster and lie back onto it. Make sure there is no gap between your pelvis and the bolster to ensure optimal lumbar support and help open your sternal area.
- Rest your knees on the second bolster and place your heels on the two vertical bricks (fig. 3.11).
- Adjust the blanket under your head, rolling its outer edges along the sides of your neck, your head, and your outer shoulders to provide complete support.

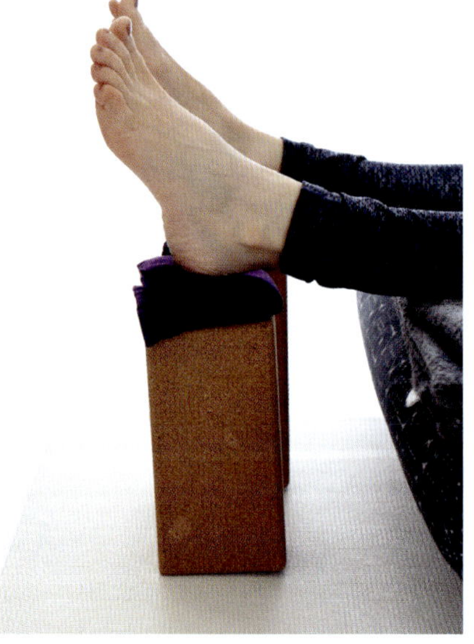

FIGURE 3.11 Feet supported on cork bricks with padding underneath to reduce pressure on the heels at rest or with bent legs in Salamba Navasana.

- Rest your hands gently on your abdomen and support your elbows with a blanket wrapped snugly around your arms (fig. 3.9).
- Cover your legs with a blanket, place an eye pillow over your eyes, and relax in this position for 20–25 minutes.

If You Feel Discomfort in Your Lower Back

- Place an additional standard-fold blanket under your seat to reduce the arch from floor to bolster.

GUIDING STUDENTS THROUGH RELAXATION

During the practice, you can use the following guidance to help students relax deeply and connect with the pose:

- Breathe naturally through your nose, allowing each inhale and exhale to flow with ease. Begin by focusing your attention on your heels. With each exhale, feel your heels dropping into the support. Trust in the stability of the bricks. As you exhale, notice your shins softening and your thighs releasing any tension.
- Gently shift your awareness upward to your face. Smooth the skin of your forehead outward toward your temples. Pay special attention to the space between your eyebrows and allow any tension there to melt away. Relax the outer muscles of your jaw and the root of your tongue, letting them soften completely. Take a moment to notice the profound sense of peace settling in your face. Let this sense of ease travel down into your neck and chest.
- Bring your focus to your belly. With each inhale, notice your belly expand slightly. With each exhale, feel it gently soften, creating a rhythm of relaxation and release.
- Place your attention on the contact between your hands and your belly. Imagine this point of contact as a bridge connecting your outer awareness to your inner self. Quietly ask yourself: "What do I need in this situation that has made me so angry?"
- Acknowledge the emotion linked to your unmet needs. If you can, name the emotion: Is it sadness, fear, shame, pain, or rage? Notice where in your body this emotion resides.
- Notice the physical sensations of this emotion without judgment.

- Stay present with these sensations, offering yourself full empathy. Gradually, you may notice a sense of relaxation beginning to emerge, gently replacing the tension.
- Throughout this process, be kind and compassionate with yourself. Treat yourself with the same care and understanding you would offer a dear friend.

TRANSITIONING OUT OF THE POSE

- As your relaxation comes to an end, gently bring your awareness back to your surroundings by taking slow, deep breaths.
- When you feel ready, slowly turn your knees inward, and with an exhale, gently press your lower back gently against the bolster.
- Take another deep breath in, and on the exhale, bend one knee, then the other, placing your feet on the bolster.
- Inhale, and as you exhale, roll onto your side on the bolster, letting your eye bag softly fall to the floor.
- When you feel ready, exhale slowly as you return to a seated position, supporting yourself with your hands.

Bhishmasana (Bed of Arrows Pose)

15–20 MINUTES

While the use of twelve bricks may seem excessive, practicing Bhishmasana, a restorative variation of Savasana, offers unique benefits that make it worth exploring. Inspired by the Mahabharata's character Bhishma, who lay on a bed of arrows, this pose involves elevating the body using bricks, allowing air to circulate underneath. This setup cools the body and creates a sensation of lightness, which can be particularly beneficial when coping with intense frustration. The firmness of the bricks also provides a distinctive sense of grounding. If you don't have enough bricks, you can opt for Salamba Savasana as an alternative (fig. 2.9).

CONTRAINDICATION

After the first trimester of pregnancy, it is recommended to practice Side-Lying Savasana on your left side (fig. 4.20).

PROPS NEEDED

1 yoga mat, 12 bricks, 1 blanket, 1 eye pillow

SETTING UP THE POSE

Arrange the bricks as follows, as shown in fig. 3.12:

- Gather twelve yoga bricks of uniform thickness and material.
- At the top of your yoga mat, place one brick widthwise to support the base of your skull.

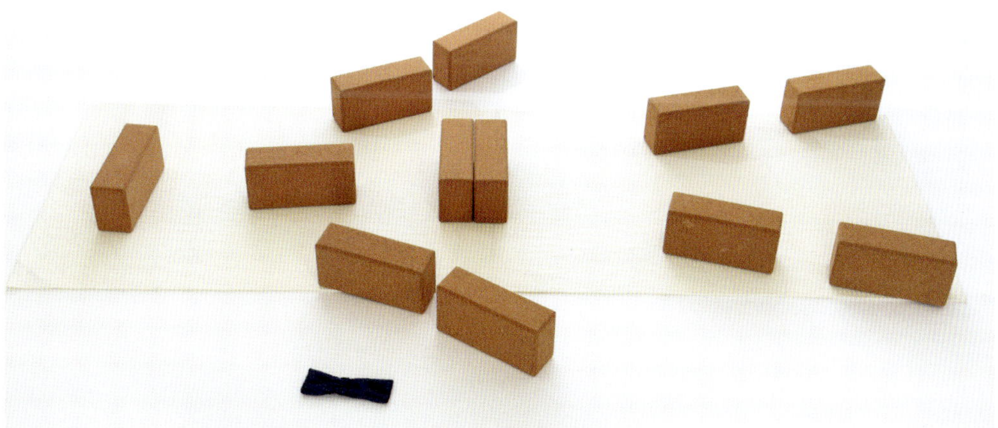

FIGURE 3.12 Setup for Bhishmasana with twelve cork bricks and an eye pillow, designed to elevate and cradle the body at multiple points: head, upper back, pelvis, legs, and arms.

- Position another brick lengthwise along the midline of your body to rest between your shoulder blades.
- Place two bricks widthwise to be under your pelvis for support.
- For each leg, position one brick to go under each knee, ensuring one half supports your thigh and the other half supports your calf. Place one brick to go under each foot to support your heels and the back of your ankles.
- For each arm, place one brick to go under each elbow and one brick under each hand.

Get into position:

- Sit on the bricks designated for your pelvis, then slowly recline, aligning your spine along the bricks.
- Adjust the brick under your head to support the occipital area, ensuring your neck remains neutral.
- Extend your legs, resting your knees on the respective bricks. Ensure each brick supports both your thigh and calf as described earlier.
- Place your feet on the designated bricks, allowing them to relax.
- Extend your arms with palms facing up, resting your elbows and hands on the bricks.
- Ensure your body is symmetrically aligned along your torso (fig. 3.13).
- Cover yourself with a blanket for warmth, close your eyes, and place an eye pillow over them.

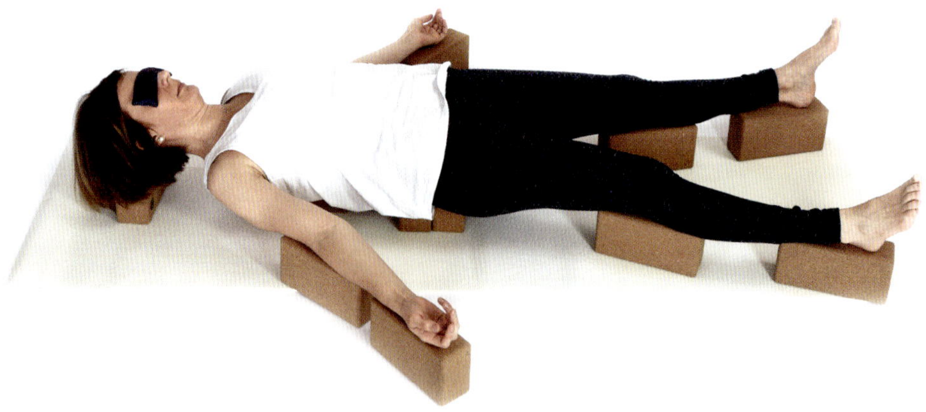

FIGURE 3.13 Audrey demonstrates Bhishmasana using twelve cork bricks placed under the head, upper back, arms, pelvis, knees, and ankles to promote deep rest and even support.

GUIDING STUDENTS THROUGH RELAXATION

During the practice, you can use the following guidance to help students relax deeply and connect with the pose:

- Gently let your eyes relax. Imagine your gaze softly turning inward, toward your heart. This subtle shift transforms your outward focus, your awareness of the external world, into a deep inner connection.
- Breathe naturally through your nose, slightly more deeply than usual. With each inhale and exhale, feel your ribs gently expand, creating a sense of spaciousness and ease.
- Observe the sensations of your breath as it flows in and out. Feel your collarbones lift on the inhale, while your upper back rests heavily on the bricks on the exhale.
- As you inhale, feel your breath filling and spreading through your collarbones and upper back. As you exhale, gently scan down your spine, noticing where your body connects with the bricks.
- Let your belly soften with each breath, like a calm pool that fills and drains effortlessly. Feel your pelvis resting heavily on the bricks, fully supported.
- Bring your awareness to the back of your head and gently scan downward, noticing every point of contact between the back of your body and the bricks. Feel how the props hold you, offering steady support.
- Let your arms rest effortlessly, noticing where they meet the surface below. There's no need for your shoulders, arms, or hands to do any work. They are fully supported, allowing your upper body to be carried with ease.
- Begin to feel the breath moving through your torso and belly. With each exhale, imagine it flowing gently down your legs and out through your feet, releasing any remaining tension.
- Let your body fully surrender into the support of the bricks, allowing your breath to flow freely and effortlessly.
- As you rest here, invite your entire being to embrace the stillness of the present moment.

TRANSITIONING OUT OF THE POSE

- As your practice comes to an end, gently bring your awareness back to where your body connects with the bricks as you take deep breaths.

- When you feel ready, open your eyes, bend one knee, then the other, and place your feet on the floor.
- Lift your pelvis, remove the two bricks, and rest your sitting bones on the mat.
- Place your nondominant hand under your skull and your dominant hand on the floor behind your back.
- Gently lift your head first, then press firmly into the floor with your hand to help yourself return to a seated position.

With your eyes closed, take a moment to assess your mental state. (See "Mindful Check-In" in chapter 3.) Observe the effects of this practice on your body, mind, and emotions. If you feel inclined, consider reflecting on the deep needs and emotions of the person with whom you experienced conflict. You may realize that your needs were, in fact, quite similar.

Engaging in such reflective practices can foster empathy and understanding, allowing for a more compassionate approach to conflict resolution. By acknowledging the commonality of human emotions and needs, we can navigate conflicts with greater ease and develop healthier relationships.

Restorative Yoga Sequences for Managing Anger

Additional sequences are provided here to help you manage your anger. Feel free to explore several of the following options to find the one that brings you the greatest sense of relaxation.

SEQUENCE 2

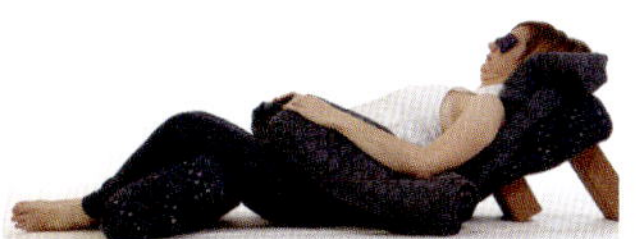

Supta Baddha Konasana (page 113)
20–30 minutes

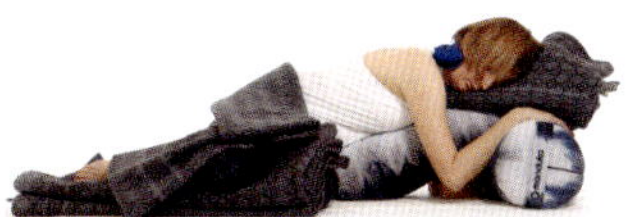

Salamba Bharadvajasana (page 53)
5 minutes each side

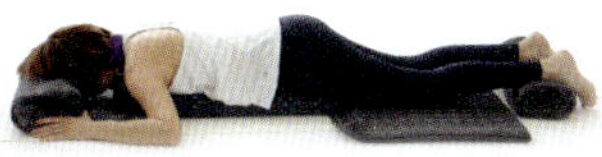

Adho Mukha Savasana with One Bolster (page 150)
15–20 minutes

SEQUENCE 3

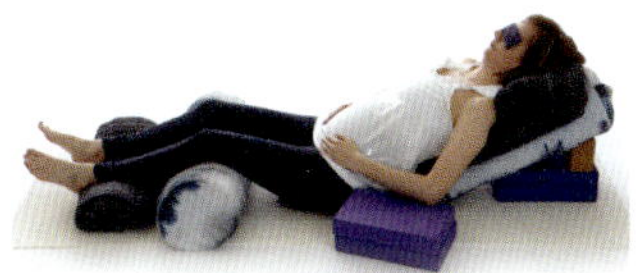

Chaise Longue Pose (page 28)
15–20 minutes

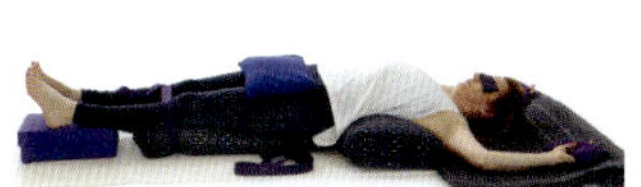

Salamba Setu Bandhasana with Straight Legs (page 94)
10–20 minutes

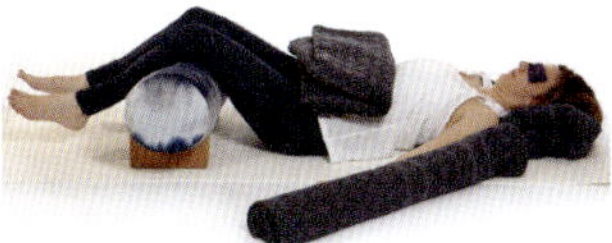

Savasana with Elevated Legs (page 187)
20 minutes

SEQUENCE 4

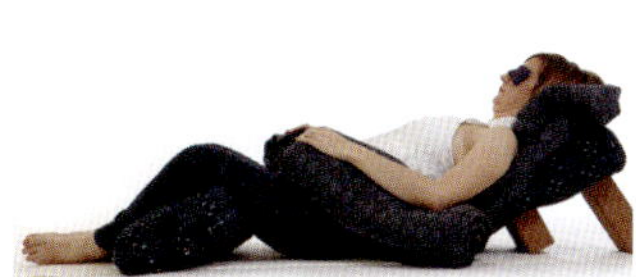

Supta Baddha Konasana (page 113)
20–30 minutes

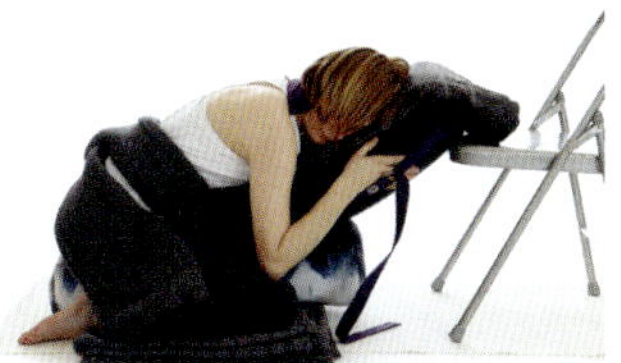

Salamba Balasana with Two Bolsters (page 116)
5 minutes each side

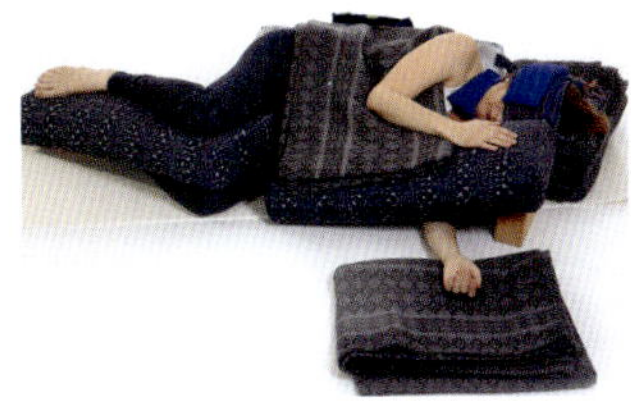

Side-Lying Savasana (page 168)
20 minutes

SEQUENCE 5 FOR ADVANCED STUDENTS

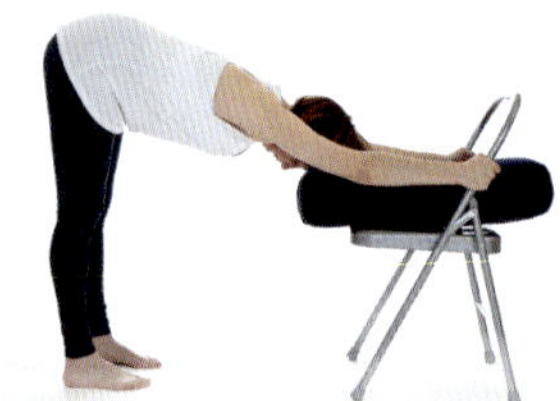

Salamba Adho Mukha Svanasana (page 180)
2–3 minutes

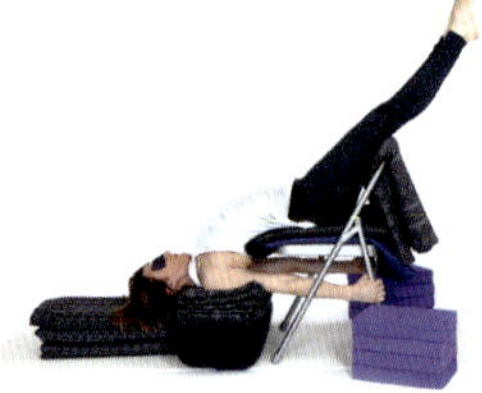

Salamba Sarvangasana (page 129)
5–10 minutes

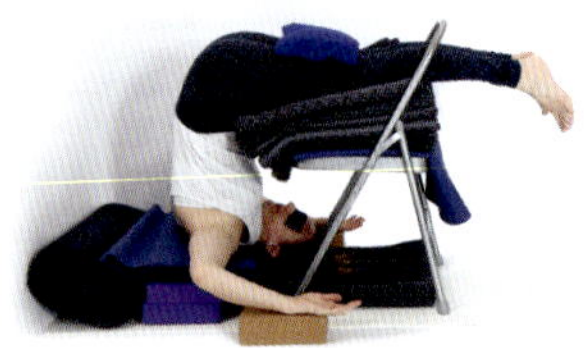

Ardha Halasana (page 141)
5–10 minutes

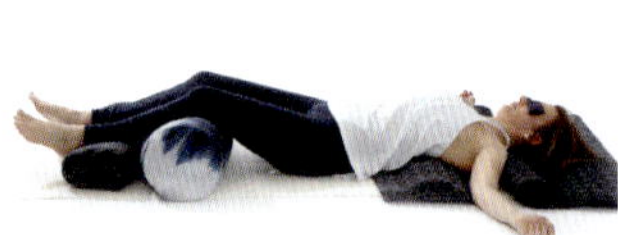

Salamba Matsyasana (page 31)
15 minutes

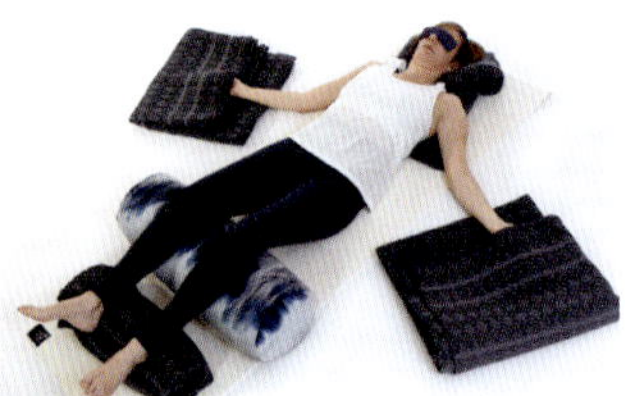

Salamba Savasana (page 41)
20 minutes

Addressing Depression

As discussed in chapter 1, excessive stimulation can overburden our nervous system, leading to a significant decrease in vagal tone. This decline impairs the vagus nerve's anti-inflammatory effects throughout the body, including the brain. The vagus nerve plays a vital role in modulating inflammation via the cholinergic anti-inflammatory pathway, which inhibits the release of pro-inflammatory cytokines. Reduced vagal activity can result in increased inflammation, contributing to various health issues, such as depression.

Depression is a widespread mental health disorder affecting 280 million people worldwide—about 3.8 percent of the global population. Notably, depression is more commonly diagnosed in women than in men. Projections suggest that by 2030 depression will become the leading cause of disease burden globally. About one-third of individuals with major depressive disorder do not experience significant improvement even after multiple courses of antidepressant treatment, highlighting the challenge of treatment-resistant depression.[6]

Depression is a complex condition that affects both the mind and the body, often leading to a pervasive sense of incapacity. Even simple tasks, such as getting out of bed, can require immense effort. Individuals may experience impaired concentration and memory, along with an intense and unusual sadness, frequently accompanied by feelings of guilt or worthlessness. The mind often dwells on past events, ruminating over what could have been done differently. Additionally, symptoms such as anxiety, insomnia, and appetite disturbances may occur.

Recent studies have also highlighted the significant role of the gut microbiota in depression. Individuals with depression often exhibit a reduced presence of beneficial bacteria such as *Coprococcus* and *Dialister* species alongside an increased abundance of *Flavonifractor*. This imbalance indicates that depression may be associated with specific changes in the gut microbiome. As discussed in chapter 1, our digestive tract communicates bidirectionally with the brain via the vagus nerve. An altered microbiome can negatively impact mood by influencing this gut-brain axis.[7]

Given the complex and multifaceted nature of depression, it is imperative to adopt a holistic approach to treatment. While antidepressants can be instrumental in initiating change, integrating complementary therapies such as Restorative Yoga can enhance long-term management of clinical depression. Restorative Yoga, in particular, has been shown to stimulate vagus nerve activity, reduce inflammation in the body and brain, and promote inward-focused awareness, all of which are beneficial in alleviating depressive symptoms.

In managing depression, altering physical states can be particularly beneficial. Practicing poses that open the chest and upper thoracic spine can counteract physical symptoms, especially what Mel Robin refers to as the tonic flexion reflex.[8] During intense sadness, the body tends to curl inward as a protective measure. Bo Forbes, a clinical psychologist and yoga therapist, describes this as the "closed heart syndrome," a pose reflecting the helplessness, despair, and self-protective withdrawal characteristic of depression.[9] In this state, the chest and heart area collapse, leading to slow and shallow breathing. The spine and shoulders round forward as if shielding the heart from further disappointment. Additional physiological symptoms include increased heart rate and output, dysfunction of internal organs, lower-back pain, abdominal tension, and posterior pelvic tilt.[10]

A 2010 Brazilian study quantitatively assessed pose and body image in individuals with major depressive disorder during depressive episodes and after treatment, comparing them to healthy controls. Findings indicated that during depressive episodes, patients exhibited increased head flexion, heightened thoracic kyphosis, a tendency toward left pelvic retroversion, and abduction of the left scapula. Notably, these postural deviations normalized following treatment, aligning with the posture of healthy individuals.[11]

Regular practice of Restorative Yoga can influence posture by modifying habitual body alignment, promoting full diaphragmatic movement, and enhancing respiratory capacity. Restorative Yoga stimulates vagus nerve activity, which can reduce inflammation in the body and brain.[12] It also enhances the ability to turn awareness inward. When the body rests and the mind remains alert, constructive internal reflection develops.[13] Focusing on physical sensations interrupts rumination over past or future events and their negative evaluations. Cultivating this skill is essential in managing depression.[14]

In addition to Restorative Yoga, daily exposure to natural light, regular physical exercise, balanced meals at consistent times, and healthy sleep patterns are important.[15] These practices combat inflammation and balance the gut microbiome, proving effective against mood disorders. To cultivate a deeper awareness of how this practice affects your body, mind, and emotions, and to enhance your interoceptive abilities, begin with assessing your mental state (see "Mindful Check-In" in chapter 3) before moving on to the sequence that follows.

Salamba Urdhva Dhanurasana (Supported Backbend) with One Blanket

10 MINUTES

Salamba Urdhva Dhanurasana with one blanket is an excellent pose to gently open the rib cage, encouraging deeper and more expansive breathing. As a mild inversion, it elevates the heart above the head, inviting a fresh perspective on life. This supported backbend also helps lengthen the spine, creating space between the vertebrae to maintain a healthy and strong back.

CONTRAINDICATIONS

- pregnancy
- menstruation
- sinusitis or nasal congestion
- gastroesophageal reflux
- spondylolysis or spondylolisthesis
- glaucoma

PROPS NEEDED

1 yoga mat, 4 blankets, 3 eye pillows

SETTING UP THE POSE

- Place a single-fold square blanket in the center of your yoga mat, ensuring the folded edge faces the top.
- Sit directly in front of the blanket on your mat.
- Slowly recline onto your back, allowing your shoulders to rest comfortably on the floor.
- Ensure that the lower tips of your shoulder blades are supported by the folded edge of the blanket. The pelvis should be only partially supported by the blanket.
- This setup allows your lower ribs to expand sideways, gently opening the chest, while your pubic bone tilts slightly downward for optimal spinal alignment.
- Another way to ensure you are on the right spot is to position your diaphragm at the center of the blanket, so both the pelvis and shoulder girdle drape off the edges. Make sure your pelvis is not fully supported by the blanket and that most of your spine does not rest directly on the floor.

- Do not place additional support under your head. This helps preserve the inversion effect of the pose and prevents unnecessary pressure on the C7 vertebra, reducing the risk of neck tension.
- On an exhale, bend your knees one at a time. Turn your feet slightly inward and let your knees rest gently against each other. This adjustment releases tension in the abdomen and lower back, promoting a sense of deep relaxation.
- Rest your arms comfortably along your sides. To increase comfort and provide a grounding sensation, you can place two single-fold square blankets under your wrists and hands, and an eye pillow on each hand (fig. 3.14).
- Cover yourself with a blanket to maintain warmth. Close your eyes and place a small eye pillow over them to foster inward focus and relaxation.
- Stay in this position for approximately 10 minutes, allowing your body to fully relax and absorb the restorative benefits of the practice.

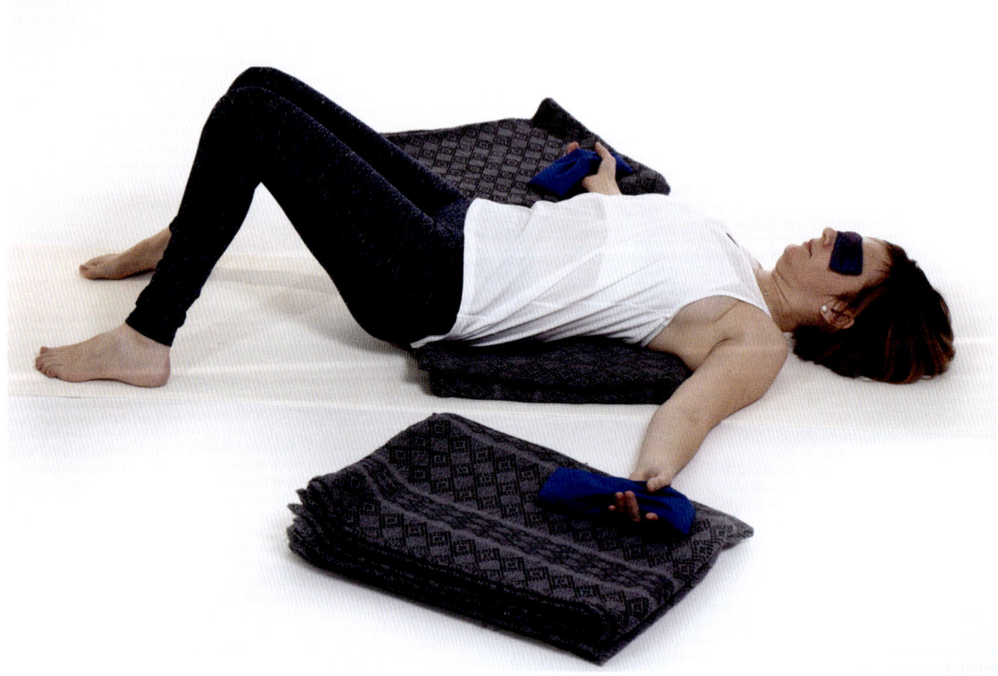

FIGURE 3.14 Audrey demonstrates Salamba Urdhva Dhanurasana with a folded blanket from the lower tips of the shoulder blades to the pelvis, allowing the tailbone to hang slightly downward. The legs are bent to support the release of the lower back.

GUIDING STUDENTS THROUGH RELAXATION

During the practice, you can use the following guidance to help students relax deeply and connect with the pose:

- Begin by breathing naturally, allowing your body to rest fully on the ground. Soften your temples, let your eyes sink gently into their sockets, and release all tension from your jaw. Allow your throat to relax, filling the space within your neck as your head sinks heavily into the earth.
- Let your shoulders release completely, dropping toward the floor.
- Imagine the earth rising up to cradle you, and notice how your arms and hands gradually become heavier with each exhale.
- Feel your knees lightly touching one another. As you exhale, allow the muscles in your legs to completely release, surrendering any effort to hold you up.
- Gently shift your awareness to your heart center. With each inhale, feel the breath expand and open the upper chest. With each exhale, feel your entire back spread even wider across the blanket.
- Imagine you could breathe through the front of your chest: air entering gently through the front of the heart, and on the exhale, flowing out through the back of the heart into the ground.
- Allow your breath to release tension and soften everything it comes into contact with. As your upper back grows more grounded, feel the throat opening and filling with ease.
- Sense the roof of your mouth widen and spread toward the sides of your cheeks and teeth, creating a space of freedom and release throughout your entire jaw and face.
- Rest here, cradled by the ground, and let your breath care for you. With each gentle inhalation and exhalation, experience a deepening sense of comfort, peace, and surrender.

TRANSITIONING OUT OF THE POSE

- When it is time to come out of the pose, gradually bring your awareness back to the sensations of the ground and the props supporting you, taking slow, mindful breaths.
- Gently slide backward until your pelvis rests on the floor. Pause here for a moment, keeping your legs bent, and allow yourself to fully settle.
- When you feel ready, roll onto your side and, with care, return to a seated position by pressing one hand near your chest into the ground while using the other hand for support.

Salamba Setu Bandhasana (Supported Bridge Pose)

15–20 MINUTES

This pose not only supports the opening of the rib cage but also invites us to connect deeply with our emotions. As humorist Steven Wright insightfully remarked, "Depression is merely anger without enthusiasm." Backbends like Salamba Setu Bandhasana play a vital role in releasing tension held within the abdomen, a region often considered the gateway to the unconscious mind. This area stores emotions and experiences that may be difficult to access through thinking alone.

By practicing this pose, we transcend the habit of filtering our emotions solely through the lens of the mind, opening instead to the raw and unfiltered experience of feeling and living fully. This embodied practice helps us cultivate a deeper awareness of our physical and emotional landscapes.

The journey of inhabiting the body is both profound and transformative. It requires patience, kindness, and self-compassion as we explore the layers of tension and emotion stored within. Yet when approached with a sense of curiosity and gentleness, Salamba Setu Bandhasana can lead to a profound sense of liberation: the joy of being present, of feeling fully alive, and of embracing the wisdom that resides within our bodies.

This pose is a bridge, not just for the spine but also for the connection of mind, body, and emotion. Through regular practice, it can foster emotional release, physical balance, and an unshakeable sense of inner harmony.

CONTRAINDICATIONS

- pregnancy
- menstruation
- sinusitis or nasal congestion
- gastroesophageal reflux
- spondylolysis and spondylolisthesis
- chronic neck pain or injuries
- retinal detachment
- glaucoma

PROPS NEEDED

1 yoga mat, 2 bolsters, 2 blankets, 2 blocks, 2 straps, 1 eye pillow, 1 sandbag

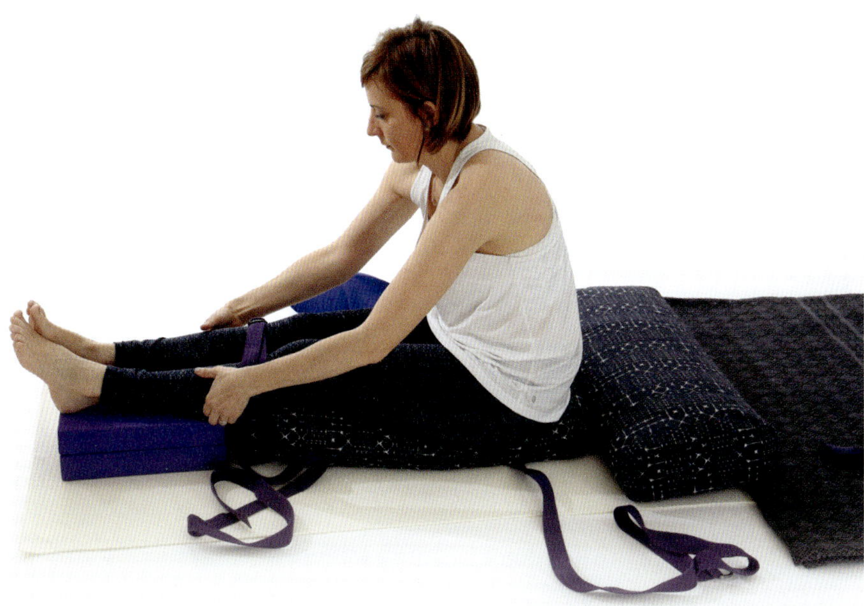

FIGURE 3.15 Audrey prepares for Salamba Setu Bandhasana by sitting on a bolster, strap around the shins for internal rotation. The strap is tight, maximum two fingers, and the buckle doesn't touch the skin.

SETTING UP THE POSE

- Place a standard blanket horizontally at the top of your yoga mat, ensuring it is smooth and evenly folded.
- Directly below the blanket, position a bolster widthwise, ensuring it is flush with the edge of the blanket. Below this bolster, place a second bolster perpendicularly to form a T shape.
- At the base of the second bolster, position two yoga blocks to comfortably support your heels.
- Place two straps under the second bolster: one for securing your shins and the other for stabilizing your upper thighs. This will help create a sense of grounding and alignment during the pose.
- Lie back onto the bolsters so that the back of your head rests comfortably on the blanket. Allow your shoulders to gently hang off the first bolster without touching the floor. This prevents the C7 vertebra at the base of your neck from pressing into the ground, which could cause tension in the neck and difficulty breathing.
- Position your diaphragm at the center of the first bolster to ensure optimal chest opening and support.

- If the chest opening feels too intense, place an additional blanket under your shoulders and head for extra support. The goal is to feel comfortably supported without any strain on your back. Remember, even a gentle chest opening is beneficial, particularly as a counterbalance to the rounded pose commonly adopted during prolonged sitting. Gradually easing into the pose prevents overstimulation of the nervous system and ensures a soothing experience.
- Extend your legs and rotate your shins inward so that your big toes touch. Secure the strap firmly around your shins to maintain this alignment, which supports the backbend (fig. 3.15).
- Buckle the second strap firmly over your body, ensuring it lies across the greater trochanters (the bony points at the top of your thighs near the hips). This belt helps your pelvis relax fully. For an added sense of grounding, you can place a sandbag over this strap.
- Cover yourself with a blanket for warmth.
- Position your arms in one of two ways:
    - **cactus shape**: Place your arms above your head in a cactus position (fig. 3.16). For added comfort, slightly elevate your hands by tucking a single-fold square blanket under them.
    - **alongside the body**: Rest your arms along your sides (fig. 3.17), with your palms facing upward.
- Enhance your sense of grounding by placing an eye pillow in the palms of your hands.
- Close your eyes and gently rest an eye pillow over them.
- Stay in this position for 15–20 minutes, allowing your body to fully relax and absorb the restorative benefits of the pose.

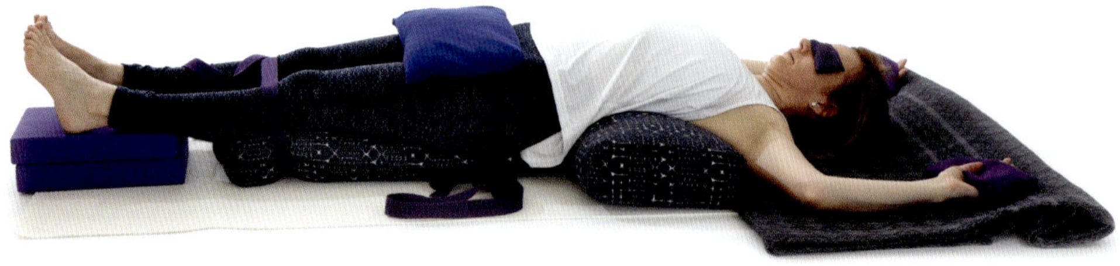

FIGURE 3.16 Audrey demonstrates Salamba Setu Bandhasana with the pelvis and rib cage supported by T-shaped bolsters, with legs and hips strapped, and a sandbag on the hips to provide grounding stability.

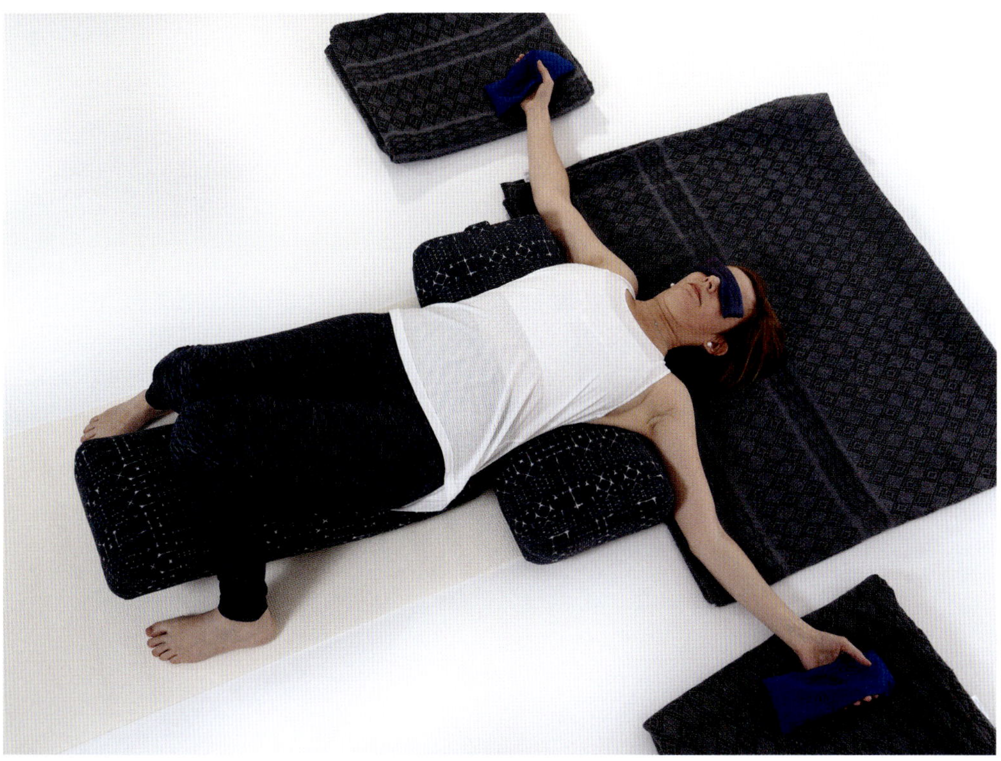

FIGURE 3.17 Audrey demonstrates a variation of Salamba Setu Bandhasana with bent legs, knees together, feet turned in, and arms supported by blankets on a T-shaped bolster setup.

Alternative Version with Bent Legs

- Instead of extending your legs, bend your knees and let them rest gently against each other. This position helps release tension in your lower back, promoting a sense of ease and relaxation.
- Rest your arms comfortably alongside your body. For added support, place single-fold square blankets under your wrists and hands. To deepen the sense of grounding, you can also place an eye pillow in the palms of your hands.
- Cover yourself with a blanket to stay warm. Close your eyes and gently place a small eye pillow over them.
- Stay in this version for 8–10 minutes, as it offers less overall support.

GUIDING STUDENTS THROUGH RELAXATION

During the practice, you can use the following guidance to help students relax deeply and connect with the pose:

- Start by focusing on your breath, gently lengthening your inhale and exhale. As you breathe more slowly, allow yourself to fully surrender into the support of the props, feeling completely held.
- Silently affirm to yourself: "This is a moment of suffering and difficulty." Repeat this phrase softly in your mind several times, allowing its meaning to settle within you. This acknowledgment helps you recognize and validate your current experience.
- Gently remind yourself: "All human beings experience moments of suffering." This helps you feel connected, reminding you that you are not alone in your challenges.
- As you continue breathing steadily through your nose, shift your awareness to your body. Slowly scan from head to toe, noticing any areas of tension, discomfort, or emotional pain. You may notice this sensation in your chest, abdomen, or another part of your body.
- Visualize your breath as a gentle, healing light. With each inhale, imagine this light flowing into areas of suffering, bringing warmth, compassion, and care. With each exhale, imagine creating space within those areas. Allow this process to feel nurturing and effortless.
- As you continue this practice, silently offer yourself kind and affirming thoughts, such as:
    - "May I find peace."
    - "I am worthy of care and kindness."
    - "It's okay to feel what I'm feeling."

  These affirmations deepen self-compassion and support emotional healing.
- Stay in this nurturing space for as long as it feels comfortable. Allow the breath to guide you. Let your breath and the support of the props cradle you, bringing comfort and ease.

TRANSITIONING OUT OF THE POSE

- When it is time to come out of the pose, begin by reconnecting with the space around you.
- Take slow, deep breaths, allowing yourself to gently transition from stillness.
- Remove the eye pillow and gently open your eyes.

- With care, remove the weight from your pubic bone.
- If possible, slowly slide backward to release yourself from the straps, allowing your pelvis to rest fully on the ground.
- Bend your legs and place your feet flat on the mat.
- When you feel ready, roll onto your side.
- Take three slow steady breaths, pausing to ground yourself. On your next exhale, use your hands for support as you gradually return to a seated position.

Self-Compassion and Restorative Yoga

When caring for others, we readily offer kindness, patience, and love. Yet, extending these same qualities to ourselves often feels much more challenging. Restorative Yoga provides a sanctuary for the body to completely relax, the nervous system to find balance, and the mind to shift from rumination to observation. This practice not only facilitates physical relaxation but also fosters the cultivation of self-compassion.

Research indicates that self-compassion practices have a profound positive impact on emotional well-being, particularly in alleviating depressive states. According to Kristin Neff, psychologist and author of *Self-Compassion: The Proven Power of Being Kind to Yourself*, self-compassion reduces depression, lowers cortisol levels, increases heart rate variability, and enhances emotional resilience.[16]

By integrating self-compassion into your Restorative Yoga practice, you create a nurturing environment for healing and growth. This combination allows you to treat yourself with the same kindness and understanding that you readily offer to others, promoting a balanced and compassionate approach to your own well-being.

Swaddled Savasana (Corpse Pose)

20–25 MINUTES

Swaddling is an ancient practice that involves wrapping a newborn in a cloth or blanket to provide comfort and help them fall asleep. This practice mimics the feeling of being fully enveloped in the womb, bringing a sense of calm and reassurance to the baby. Swaddled Savasana re-creates this effect using several blankets, offering us the opportunity to reconnect with deeply rooted sensations of maternal protection. Engaging in Swaddled Savasana can provide numerous benefits:

- **deep relaxation**: The gentle pressure from the blankets can help soothe the nervous system, promoting a state of deep relaxation.
- **stress reduction**: Similar to the effects of weighted blankets, swaddling can reduce feelings of stress and anxiety, fostering a sense of security.
- **enhanced sleep quality**: By calming the mind and body, this practice may improve sleep quality and alleviate insomnia.
- **muscle relaxation**: The supportive wrapping allows muscles to release tension, aiding in overall physical relaxation.

By practicing Swaddled Savasana, you can experience a profound sense of comfort and tranquility, reconnecting with innate feelings of safety and warmth.

CONTRAINDICATIONS

After the first trimester of pregnancy, it is recommended to practice Side-Lying Savasana on your left side (fig. 4.20).

PROPS NEEDED

1 yoga mat, 5 blankets, 1 eye pillow

SETTING UP THE POSE

- Sit on your yoga mat with your legs extended in front of you.
- Fold a standard blanket into two layers and place it horizontally at the top of your mat. The higher layer should support your head, with the thickest edge placed under the C7 vertebra for optimal support, while the lower layer, with its thinnest edge, supports the top of your shoulder blades. Roll the blanket's edges gently to cradle the sides of your neck, head, and outer shoulders for full support.

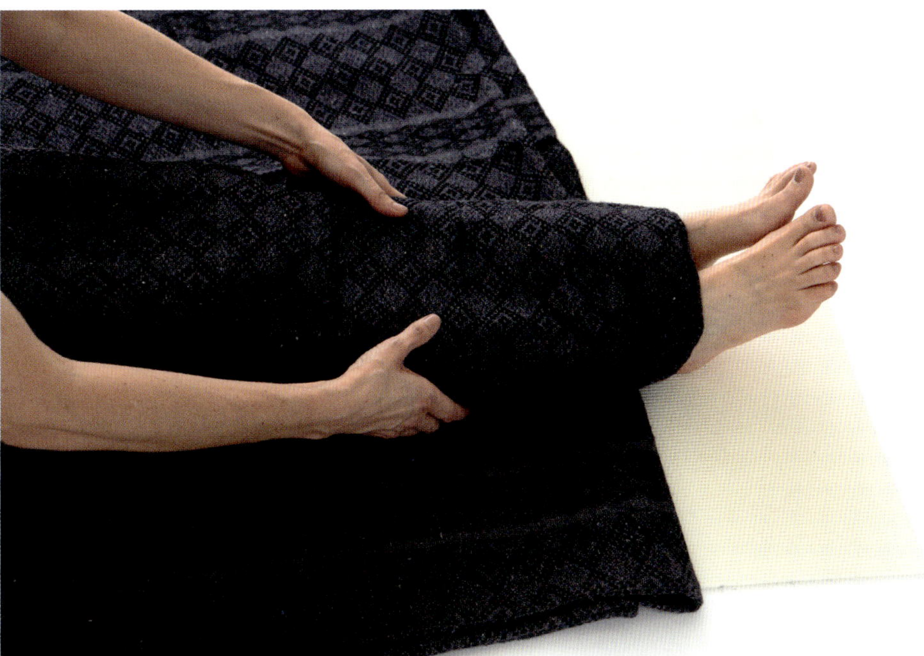

FIGURE 3.18 The legs being wrapped in a firm swaddle in Swaddled Savasana using a standard blanket unfolded once, with slight internal rotation to prevent outward rolling.

- Drape a standard-fold blanket over your lower legs, covering your ankles and knees. Rotate your legs inward gently to align them in a neutral position. Wrap the blanket snugly around your legs, tucking the edges firmly under the sides to keep them securely in place. This alignment mirrors Tadasana (Mountain Pose) and can alleviate sacroiliac discomfort (fig. 3.18).
- Place another standard-fold blanket over your feet, ensuring they are comfortably covered and warm.
- Lay a standard-fold blanket over your abdomen and thighs, extending it to your knees. Similarly, wrap yourself by tucking the blanket's edges along both sides of your body, securing it snugly to maintain hip alignment and promote a sense of stability (fig. 3.19).
- Lie on your back, positioning your head on the prepared blanket. Adjust the blanket to cradle your neck and head comfortably.
- Place another standard-fold blanket over your torso. Position your arms at a minimum 45-degree angle from your body. Ensure your arms are not too close to your sides, as this could restrict the movement of your ribs and limit your breathing. Rest your elbows on the ground, with your palms facing upward or inward toward your body.

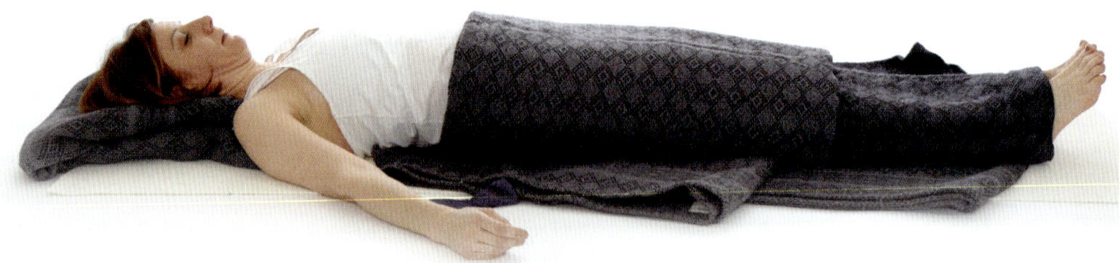

FIGURE 3.19 After supporting her head with a blanket and swaddling her legs in Swaddled Savasana, Audrey added a second standard blanket, unfolded once, to wrap from her thighs up to just below the floating ribs.

- Make sure no part of your body is left uncovered. Place an eye pillow over your eyes and securely wrap each arm to ensure they do not rest directly on the ground (fig. 3.20).
- Settle into the pose and relax in silence for 20–25 minutes.

GUIDING STUDENTS THROUGH RELAXATION

During the practice, you can use the following guidance to help students relax deeply and connect with the pose:

- Begin by taking several deep, soothing breaths. With each inhale, invite relaxation into your body. With each exhale, let go of any tension or discomfort.

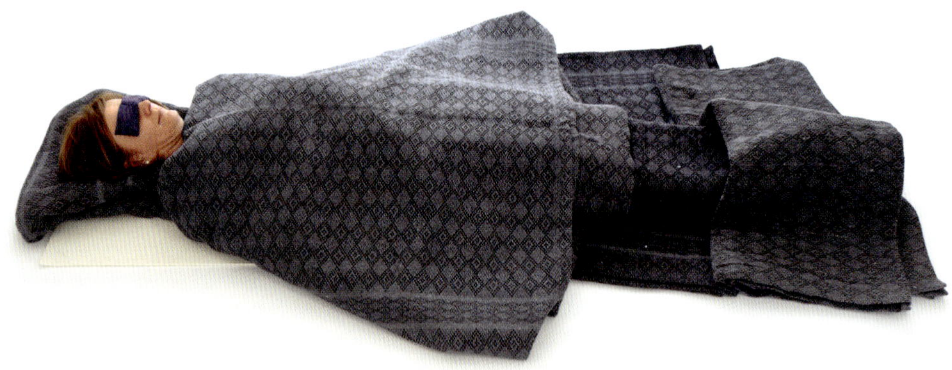

FIGURE 3.20 Audrey demonstrates the final setup for Swaddled Savasana with the whole body wrapped in blankets, arms wide open to support the breath, and an eye pillow for relaxation.

- Slowly bring your attention to the crown of your head and begin a gentle body scan. Gradually move your awareness down—through your face, neck, shoulders, arms, torso, hips, and legs—all the way to the tips of your toes. Pause whenever you notice tension, discomfort, or resistance.
- When you encounter tension, resist the urge to analyze or think about it. Instead, simply acknowledge its presence. Imagine holding this tension gently, as if comforting a dear friend.
- Picture your breath as a soft, nurturing wave, surrounding the area of resistance with warmth and compassion.
- If it feels natural, silently say to the area of tension: "I see you. I hear you." Offer it care and kindness, letting it know that it has been noticed and understood.
- Observe any changes or sensations in that part of your body. Perhaps the tension feels lighter, softer, or less defined. Or it may remain unchanged, which is equally okay. Simply hold space for whatever arises, without judgment.
- After scanning your entire body, return to your breath. Notice how your body feels as a whole: grounded, supported, and at ease. Rest here in the comforting embrace of Savasana.

TRANSITIONING OUT OF THE POSE

- At the end of the practice, bring your awareness to the points of contact between your body and the ground.
- On an exhale, gently press your lower back into the floor and carefully unwrap yourself from the blankets.
- Bend one knee, then the other.
- Slowly roll onto the side of your choice and rest here for a few breaths.
- When you feel ready, return to a seated position, pressing one hand near your chest into the floor while using the other for support.
- With your eyes still closed, take a few moments to notice the effects of this sequence on your body, mind, and emotions. Observe any changes with curiosity and without judgment.

Restorative Yoga Sequences for Managing Depression

Other sequences can also be effective in managing depressive states. When experiencing significant lethargy, shorter durations in each pose and more frequent transitions between them may provide greater relief and energy. Experiment with the following sequences to discover the one that aligns best with your needs and current state. Allow yourself the freedom to adapt and explore until you find what feels most supportive.

SEQUENCE 2

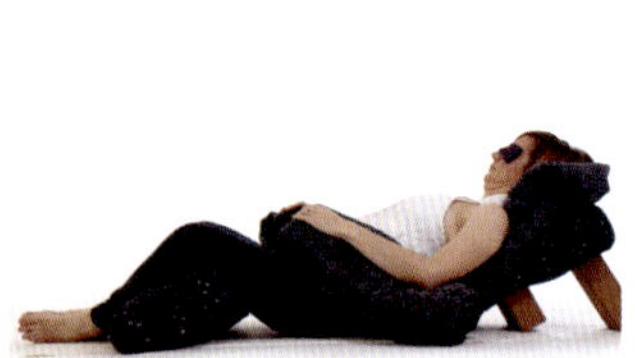

Supta Baddha Konasana
(page 113)
15–20 minutes

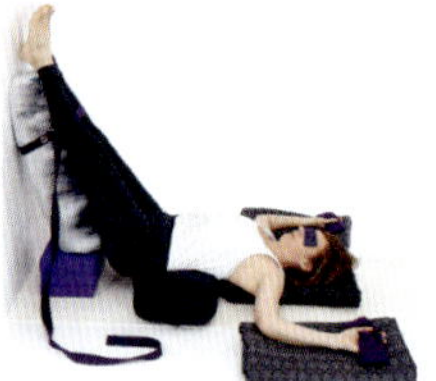

Viparita Karani
(page 183)
10–15 minutes

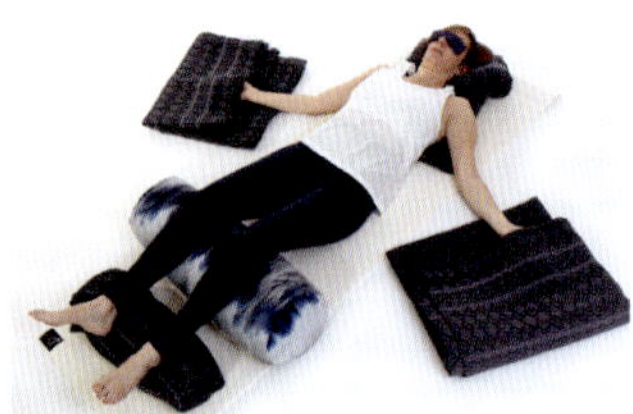

Salamba Savasana
(page 41)
20–25 minutes

SEQUENCE 3

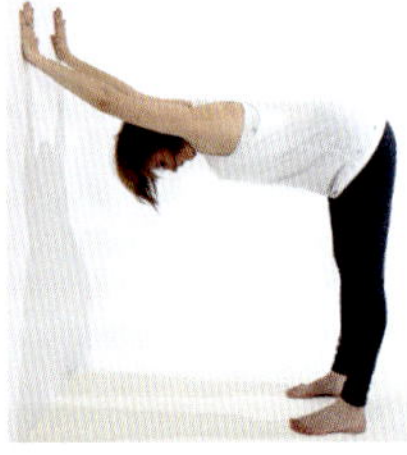

Ardha Svanasana
(page 158)
2–3 minutes

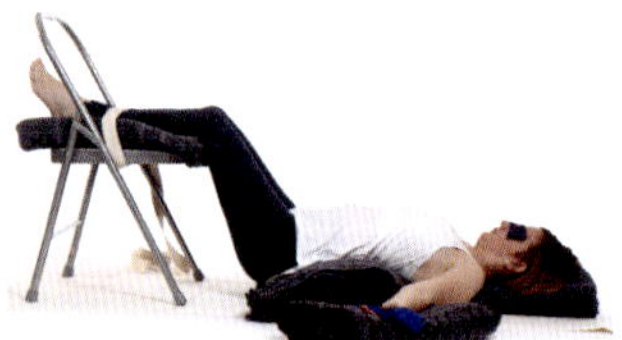

Ardha Viparita Karani
(page 56)
15–20 minutes

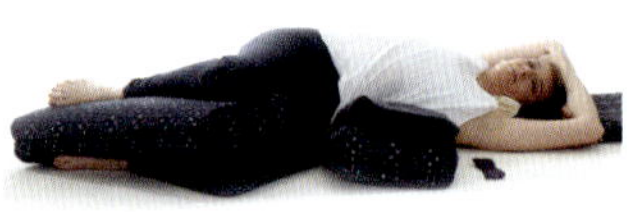

Salamba Jathara Parivartanasana (page 35)
3–5 minutes each side

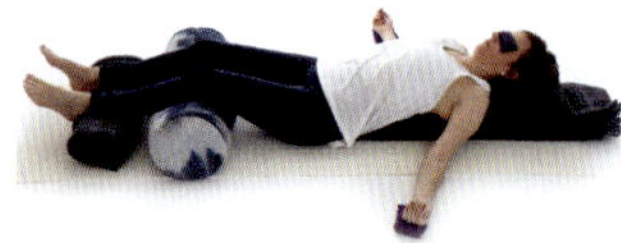

Savasana for Pranayama with Sama Vritti (page 60)
20–25 minutes

SEQUENCE 4

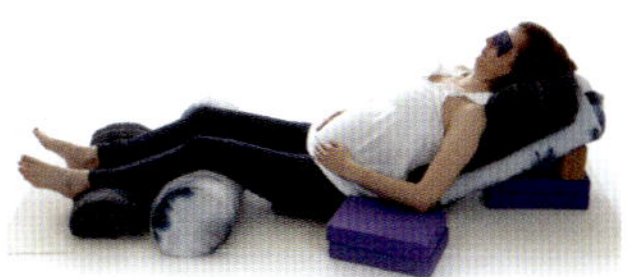

Chaise Longue Pose (page 28)
15–20 minutes

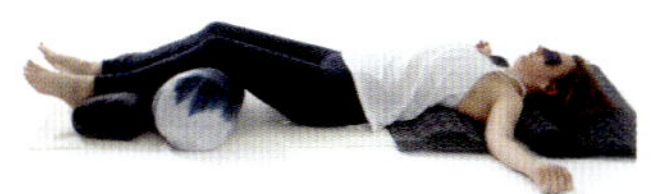

Salamba Matsyasana (page 31)
10–15 minutes

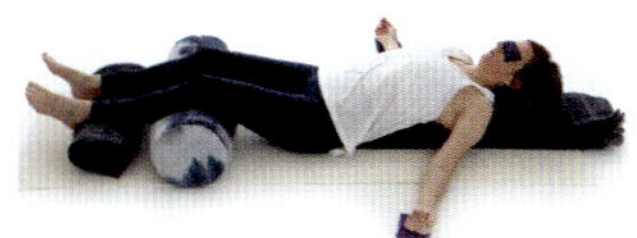

Savasana for Pranayama with Sama Vritti (page 60)
20–25 minutes

SEQUENCE 5 FOR ADVANCED STUDENTS

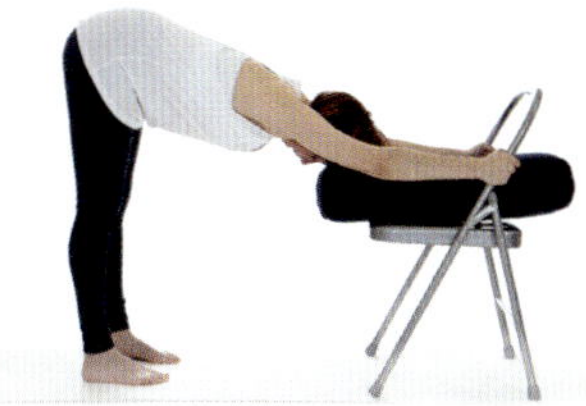

Salamba Adho Mukha Svanasana (page 180)
2–3 minutes

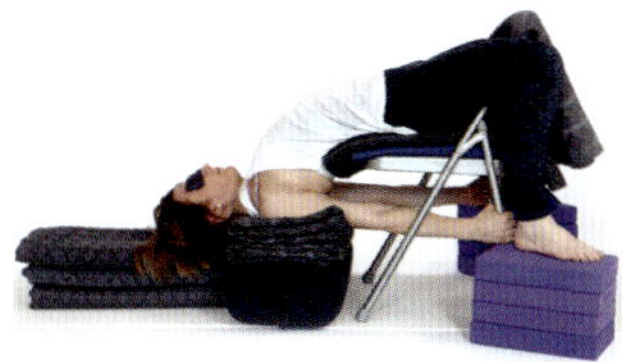

Salamba Urdhva Dhanurasana with a Chair (page 135)
5 minutes

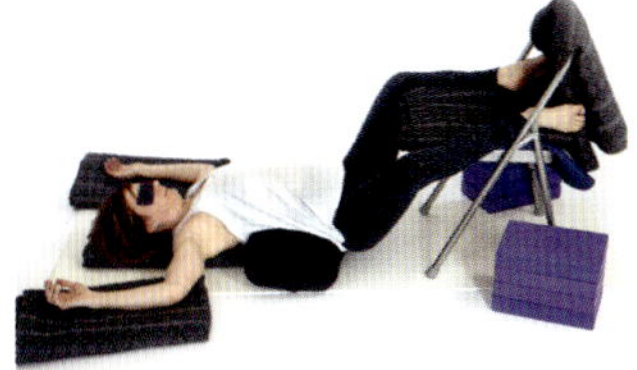

Viparita Baddha Konasana (page 138)
15–20 minutes

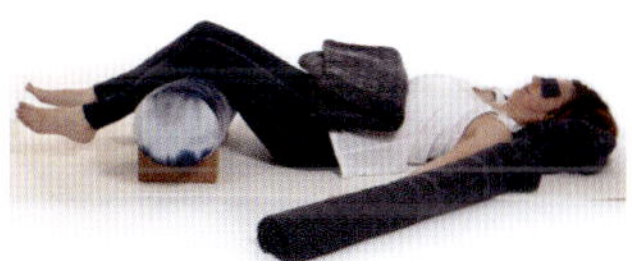

Savasana with Elevated Legs (page 187)
20 minutes

CHAPTER 4

Nurturing Well-Being Through Hormonal Shifts

Hormones are more than just chemical messengers. They shape how we feel, how we relate to the world, and how we experience major life transitions. For individuals with ovaries, hormonal shifts are particularly influential. From the first menstrual cycle to menopause and beyond, these internal tides affect not only physical health but also emotional well-being and resilience.

This chapter explores how stress impacts hormonal balance and how practices like Restorative Yoga can offer supportive tools for navigating menstruation, fertility, pregnancy, and menopause. By learning to support the body's natural rhythms, we can foster a greater sense of ease and vitality throughout all phases of life.

Hormones and Emotional Sensitivity

Research has shown that individuals assigned female at birth are approximately twice as likely to experience depression as those assigned male. One explanation comes from neuroscience. According to Dr. Louann Brizendine, founder of the Women's Mood and Hormone Clinic at the University of California, San Francisco, this increased sensitivity can be traced back to adolescence. The activation of the hypothalamic-pituitary-ovarian axis sends waves of estrogen and progesterone through the body and brain. These surges continue throughout life—fluctuating with each menstrual cycle, pregnancy, postpartum phase, and finally, the transition into menopause.[1]

Each of these hormonal seasons carves new neural pathways. They don't just change our bodies: They change our minds and brains. These changes aren't inherently negative. They reflect the body's natural wisdom. But when the demands of life outpace our capacity to adapt, these transitions can become sources of suffering. To respond more compassionately to these shifts, we can turn to two ancient healing traditions: Ayurveda and Traditional Chinese Medicine (TCM). Both systems offer a more nuanced understanding of the body—one that sees hormonal changes as expressions of deeper energetic forces.

Yin and Yang: The Energies Behind Hormones

In both Ayurveda and TCM, life is governed by two complementary energies:

- **yang**: the energy of movement, transformation, and action
- **yin**: the energy of rest, nourishment, and stability

In the body, every structure contains these two polarities. Yang animates and activates while yin sustains and soothes. This energetic balance is essential not only for physical health but also for emotional regulation. Yin corresponds to fluids and tissues like blood, lymph, and interstitial fluids. Yang is the spark that moves energy through the system. Without yin, yang burns out. Without yang, yin becomes stagnant.

In TCM, the free flow of qi, or prana in Ayurveda, reflects this balance. When qi flows smoothly, the body feels well resourced and the mind is at ease. But when yin or yang becomes deficient or dominant, imbalances occur. These imbalances often manifest as fatigue, irritability, insomnia, or hormonal symptoms like irregular cycles, premenstrual syndrome (PMS), and hot flashes.

HORMONES AS EXPRESSIONS OF YIN AND YANG

Sex hormones like estrogen and progesterone are considered expressions of yin. They nourish, moisten, and soften. Estrogen in particular is called "the yin within the yin."[2] It supports skin, bones, cognitive function, and emotional resilience. Stress hormones like adrenaline and cortisol embody yang energy. They stimulate the body's alert systems, heighten vigilance, and prepare us for danger. They're helpful in small doses. But when stress becomes chronic, these yang hormones dominate. And without enough yin to buffer their effects, the body enters a cycle of depletion.

Many modern hormonal issues—fatigue, anxiety, PMS, thyroid disorders, fertility challenges—can be viewed through this lens: too much yang, not enough yin.

SUPPORTING THE YIN OF HORMONAL BALANCE

Estrogen and progesterone play a vital role in regulating mood, sleep, and emotional stability. As these hormones fluctuate, especially during midlife, symptoms like hot flashes, brain fog, and irritability may appear. This isn't a failure of the body. It's a signal that more yin is needed.

Yin can be replenished through sleep, nutrition, emotional connection, and therapeutic practices like Restorative Yoga. Restorative poses slow down the nervous system, enhance vagal tone, and support the body's ability to repair.

Research backs this up. In 2006 Judith Hanson Lasater consulted on NIH studies that showed that Restorative Yoga significantly reduced the intensity and frequency of hot flashes in menopausal participants, even those without previous yoga experience.[3]

Chronic Stress and Hormonal Depletion

When stress becomes a constant in our lives, the adrenal glands go into overdrive, producing high levels of cortisol to help the body cope. Over time, this depletes our hormonal reserves. Progesterone is often the first to be redirected, converted into cortisol to meet the body's survival demands.

This is where things get more complicated: The body can convert progesterone into estrogen, but not the other way around. So when progesterone levels drop, the body struggles to maintain a stable and healthy level of estrogen. In other words, a lack of progesterone doesn't just cause its own set of symptoms; it also makes the effects of low estrogen more pronounced.

This dynamic can create a vicious cycle. More stress leads to more cortisol, which drains the body's yin hormones, especially progesterone and estrogen. As these stores diminish, the endocrine system becomes increasingly strained, impacting everything from mood and memory to digestion, sleep, and immune function.

Recovery and Resilience

The good news is that the body is always seeking balance. Hormones like DHEA, oxytocin, and prolactin offer a counterbalance to cortisol. They support connection, tenderness, and repair, and they can be encouraged through practices that foster safety, presence, and rest. Restorative Yoga is one such practice. By gently activating the parasympathetic nervous system, it gives the body permission to rebuild. Over time, this replenishes yin and reduces the dominance of yang.

A New Hormonal Literacy

The wisdom of the body is cyclical, not linear. Hormones ebb and flow like the tides. Yet in a culture that prizes speed, productivity, and constant output, we're taught to override these natural rhythms. But the body remembers.

Learning to respect hormonal shifts as part of a broader energetic landscape allows us to respond with compassion rather than control. When we listen deeply, slow down, and create supportive environments, we open the door to healing—not only physically, but emotionally and spiritually.

Hormonal health is not just about lab values or symptoms. It's about how we live in our bodies, how we honor our energy, and how we attune to our needs and the seasons of our inner world. This is the heart of Restorative Yoga: a practice rooted in restoration, presence, and wholeness.

In addition to balancing the nervous system and replenishing yin energy, Restorative Yoga also supports hormonal equilibrium—through the power of stillness, a sense of safety, and the therapeutic effects of specific poses.

How Do Restorative Yoga Poses Influence Hormonal Balance?

The pituitary gland, situated at the base of the brain, plays a key role in hormonal regulation and is divided into two main sections:

- The anterior lobe secretes hormones that support reproductive functions in individuals with ovaries, including regulation of the menstrual cycle and ovulation.
- The posterior lobe regulates secretions and nourishes the smooth muscles of the uterus, enhancing its overall functionality.

Certain Restorative Yoga poses are particularly effective in stimulating these functions:

- **Inverted poses** stimulate the pituitary gland, supporting hormonal regulation.
- **Forward bends** enhance blood flow to the pelvic organs, delivering fresh, oxygenated blood and alleviating menstrual discomfort.

Ancient Indian texts offer another perspective on how asanas influence hormonal balance, emphasizing the importance of consciously working with two fundamental energies in the body: prana and *apana*, which are essential for both physical and mental health:

- **prana**: Often associated with masculine energy, prana resides above the diaphragm and tends to move upward. It governs the heart and respiratory system.
- **apana**: Linked to feminine energy, apana resides below the diaphragm and tends to move downward. It governs the abdominal, pelvic, and lower body organs.

Achieving hormonal balance involves identifying which energy to cultivate and practicing poses that align with this goal:

- **Inversions** increase apana, calming the mind and stimulating the abdominal organs, including the reproductive organs.
- **Seated forward bends** and **supine poses** harmonize both prana and apana, quieting and relaxing the abdominal organs.

For example, if you are struggling with infertility or experiencing menopausal hot flashes, focus on increasing apana through inversions. If you are menstruating or pregnant, prioritize calming poses that harmonize prana and apana to avoid overstimulation. By understanding the unique benefits of Restorative Yoga poses, practitioners can effectively support hormonal balance and address specific needs at different stages of life.

Before beginning your practice, take a moment to assess your mental state. (See "Mindful Check-In" in chapter 3.) Pausing for reflection before and after your Restorative Yoga session heightens awareness of the effects of poses on your body, mind, and emotions. Cultivating this mindfulness can inspire consistent and fulfilling practice.

During Menstruation

Smooth and trouble-free menstruation depends on the harmonious functioning of the ovaries, pituitary gland, and hypothalamus. The hypothalamus works closely with the pituitary gland to regulate ovarian activity, ensuring a regular menstrual cycle. As previously discussed, practicing inversions outside menstruation can be particularly beneficial for stimulating the pituitary gland and promoting hormonal balance.

However, during menstruation, it is essential to adapt yoga practices to align with the body's natural rhythms. The focus should shift toward calming and restorative poses, such as gentle forward bends and 45-degree-angle poses while avoiding inversions. Inversions, which place the uterus or abdominal area above the heart, can disrupt the natural flow of menstrual energy. Similarly, poses that elevate the legs above heart level should also be avoided to prevent interference with the body's natural processes.

The Science Behind Avoiding Inversions During Menstruation

The rationale for avoiding inversions during menstruation can be understood from both Western and Eastern perspectives:

- **From a Western viewpoint:** Inversions cause the uterus to shift toward the head due to gravity, potentially reducing or blocking the blood supply to the uterus. This may temporarily halt menstrual flow, followed by a heavier and more painful discharge.

- **From an Eastern perspective:** Inversions are believed to disrupt apana, the downward-moving energy responsible for elimination processes, including menstruation. This disruption may cause stagnation in the pelvic region, leading to similar outcomes.[4]

Considering Common Menstrual Disorders

Many people of childbearing age experience conditions such as endometriosis, a chronic gynecological condition affecting about 10 percent of those who menstruate worldwide. This number likely underestimates the prevalence due to underdiagnosis. Symptoms often include painful periods (dysmenorrhea), pain during intercourse (dyspareunia), chronic pelvic and lower-back pain, and painful bowel movements (dyschezia), which are often unresponsive to standard pain relief methods.

Endometriosis has multifactorial origins, with retrograde menstruation playing a significant role. While most menstrual blood exits the uterus through the vagina, some may flow backward through the fallopian tubes into the abdominal cavity. This retrograde flow can transport endometrial fragments or stem cells capable of establishing ectopic endometrial tissue. These tissues respond to hormonal cycles by bleeding during menstruation; however, unlike normal menstrual blood, they cannot exit the body. Consequently, the accumulation of this blood in the abdominal cavity leads to tissue damage and inflammation, contributing to the development and progression of endometriosis.

While retrograde menstruation is a key factor, not everyone with this condition develops endometriosis. Other factors, including genetic predisposition, immune system dysfunction, and environmental influences, also contribute to the pathogenesis of this disease.

During menstruation, it is crucial to practice yoga poses that support the natural downward and outward flow of menstrual blood. As cyclical beings, acknowledging this rhythm aligns with yoga's principles of self-awareness and acceptance. Menstruation should be embraced as a time for introspection, rest, and self-care.

This sequence is designed to harmonize apana, the feminine energy in the abdomen, while alleviating menstrual discomfort experienced by approximately 40 percent of people who menstruate. It is also beneficial during the days leading up to menstruation for PMS, after a miscarriage, or shortly after childbirth. Additionally, this practice may support individuals living with fibroids or endometriosis.

Supta Baddha Konasana (Reclining Bound Angle Pose)

20–25 MINUTES

Supta Baddha Konasana is an excellent starting point for a Restorative Yoga sequence during menstruation. This pose promotes deep relaxation in the pelvic region, helping to alleviate menstrual discomfort such as abdominal cramps and mood swings. Beyond its benefits during menstruation, Supta Baddha Konasana supports practitioners throughout various life stages:

- **fertility support**: By enhancing blood circulation to the pelvic area, this pose may promote reproductive health.
- **pregnancy and early labor**: The gentle opening of the hips and groin can provide comfort during pregnancy and assist in early labor by relaxing the uterus.
- **postpartum recovery**: Practicing this pose postpartum can help reduce physical and mental stress and fatigue, supporting both mothers and birthing individuals as they adjust to the demands of the postpartum period. It also improves blood flow to the abdominal organs, aiding in recovery and revitalization.
- **menopausal relief**: Regular practice may help alleviate symptoms like hot flashes and anxiety, offering comfort during menopause.

Incorporating Supta Baddha Konasana into your routine provides a sanctuary of tranquility, fostering physical ease and emotional balance during the menstrual cycle and beyond.

PROPS NEEDED

1 yoga mat, 2–3 bricks, 2 bolsters, 5 blankets, 1 eye pillow

SETTING UP THE POSE

- Place a bolster lengthwise on your yoga mat, supported by two bricks to create a 45-degree angle. Position one brick vertically under the bolster near the short end and a second brick horizontally at the middle of the bolster. This 45-degree angle setup is a variation from Chaise Longue Pose (fig. 2.5), where we used one bolster, two blocks, and a brick; Salamba Bharadvajasana (fig. 3.2), where we used two bolsters; and Salamba Navasana (see fig. 3.10), where a chair was turned upside down on the floor with a bolster resting on it. Choose the setup that best suits your needs and available props.

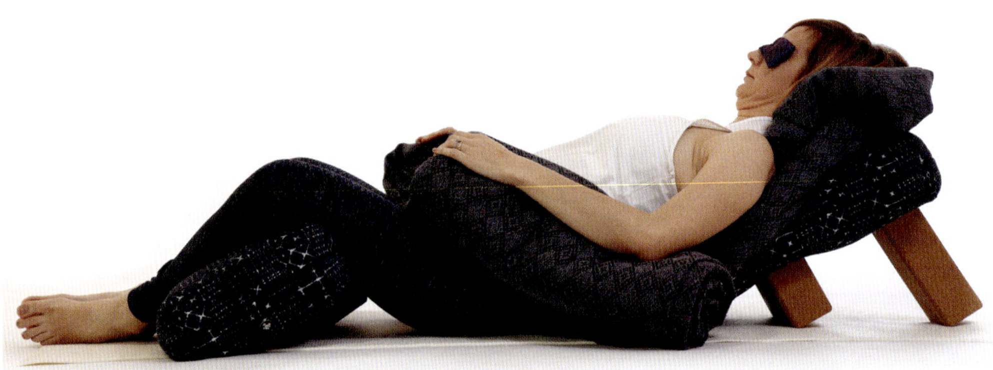

FIGURE 4.1 Audrey demonstrates Supta Baddha Konasana at a 45-degree angle. The position of the legs supports the opening of the lower lungs. The arms form a closed circle for ease and protection.

- Cover the bolster and the floor with a blanket folded in half widthwise to provide extra comfort for your back.
- At the top of the bolster, add a standard-fold blanket folded into two layers. The higher layer should support your head, with the thick edge placed under the C7 vertebra for optimal support. The lower layer, with its thin edge, supports the top of your shoulder blades.
- Sit in front of the bolster with your legs extended, and then lie back onto the bolster. Ensure there's no gap between your pelvis and the bolster to ensure optimal lumbar support and help open your sternal area.
- Bend your knees and bring the soles of your feet together, allowing your knees to fall outward into a butterfly position. Place a second bolster under your knees. If you're using a rectangular bolster (in fig. 4.1), place a brick under the bolster. Your knees should rest on the edge of the bolster. Ensure your inner thighs are relaxed and not stretched, as adequate support under the thighs is essential to avoid overstretching the anterior sacral ligaments.
- Adjust the blanket under your head, rolling its outer edges along the sides of your neck, your head, and your outer shoulders to provide complete support.
- Place one rolled blanket under each elbow, arm, and hand. Ensure your hands are higher than your elbow to help relax your shoulders.
- Cover yourself with a blanket, place an eye pillow over your eyes, and relax for 20 minutes.

If You Feel Discomfort in Your Lower Back

- Place an additional standard-fold blanket under your seat to reduce the arch from floor to bolster.

GUIDING STUDENTS THROUGH RELAXATION

During the practice, you can use the following guidance to help students relax deeply and connect with the pose:

- Feel your hands resting gently on your abdomen, receiving your breath. Take a moment to ensure you are in the most comfortable position, making any adjustments you need to feel fully supported and relaxed.
- Breathe naturally through your nose, and direct your awareness to the areas where your body contacts the props. Begin with the back of your head, noticing the soothing touch of the blanket: behind your ears, along the sides of your neck, and under your outer shoulders. Feel the entire back of your lungs and heart supported by the bolster.
- Shift your attention to your lower back, sensing the bolster perfectly following the curve of your spine. Notice where your seat meets the ground. Allow your legs to be completely held by the bolster, with your feet nestled together, supported by the ground. Let your body be fully cradled by the props, creating space for your breath to flow freely.
- Now focus on your breath. Feel the air entering your nostrils, traveling down into your expanding lungs, then rising as it gently escapes, retracing its path back out through your nostrils. Breathe naturally and stay focused on the physical sensations of your breath.
- As you rest here, let the gentle rhythm of your inhale and exhale rock you into a state of calm, each breath a soothing wave inviting you deeper into stillness.

TRANSITIONING OUT OF THE POSE

- When it is time to come out of the pose, begin by gently bringing your awareness to the sensations of contact with the ground and the props supporting your body.
- Take a deep inhale, and on your exhale, slowly bring the soles of your feet to the floor, one at a time.
- Next roll onto your side, letting the bolster continue to support you as the eye pillow gently slips away. Pause here for a moment, taking a few breaths to transition mindfully.
- When you feel ready, use your hands to support yourself as you gradually return to a seated position. Move slowly and deliberately, honoring the sense of calm and restoration cultivated during the practice.

Salamba Balasana (Supported Child Pose)

3–5 MINUTES EACH SIDE

This pose is particularly beneficial during menstruation, as the gentle pressure on the uterus helps alleviate menstrual cramps by relaxing the muscles in the pelvic region. The forward-fold position promotes a sense of grounding, which can soothe mood fluctuations commonly experienced during this time.

In addition to its physical benefits, this pose fosters a sense of support and nurturing. The use of props allows the body to fully surrender, encouraging profound relaxation and renewal.

CONTRAINDICATIONS

- **knee injuries:** Practitioners with current or recent knee injuries should avoid this pose, as it places pressure on the knee joints.
- **ankle injuries:** Those with ankle injuries should exercise caution, as the pose involves flexion of the ankles.
- **pregnancy:** After the first trimester, avoid this pose to prevent any pressure on the abdomen.

PROPS NEEDED

1 yoga mat, 2 bolsters, 1 chair or sofa, 5 blankets, 1 eye pillow

SETTING UP THE POSE

- Place a chair facing you at one end of your yoga mat. If a chair is unavailable, use the seat of a sofa. Position your yoga mat in front of the sofa to create a stable setup.
- At the opposite end of the mat, place two standard blankets widthwise to slightly lift your ankles. Tuck the thin edge under your ankle joints to reduce stiffness and provide adequate support for your feet and ankles.
- Lay a bolster lengthwise across the blankets. This bolster will serve as a seat, elevating your pelvis and reducing pressure on your knee joints.
- Prepare the second bolster and strap: loop a yoga strap lengthwise around the second bolster and secure it tightly. Adjust the strap so it is snug enough to support your hands during the pose.
- Sit astride the first bolster, with your shins resting on the blankets and your feet extending just beyond their edges. Keep your feet pointing straight back to maintain proper alignment and prevent unnecessary strain on the inner knees.

- Place one short end of the second bolster against your pubic bone and the opposite end on the seat of the chair or sofa. If the bolster is too soft, support it with yoga bricks to prevent it from sinking under your weight. The setup should create a comfortable 45-degree angle.
- Cover the second bolster with a single-fold rectangular blanket to elevate your torso slightly and provide additional padding for comfort.
- Before leaning forward, fold a blanket lengthwise three times to create a narrow strip. Place the folded blanket horizontally across your abdomen, between your lower ribs and hip bones. Ensure it's under your abdomen, not under your hips. Take both ends of the blanket and wrap them around your pelvis, similar to tying a kimono belt. Secure it with a knot at your back, providing gentle compression to relieve menstrual discomfort.
- Lean your torso forward onto the second bolster, resting comfortably. Turn your head to one side and slightly tuck your chin. Your back should curve outward in slight flexion from the base of your neck all the way to your pelvis (fig. 4.2). Ensure that the back of your neck is long and not extended. If needed, reduce the bolster's angle for better alignment.
- Place an eye pillow at the back of your neck to encourage deeper relaxation. Cover yourself with a blanket for warmth and comfort.

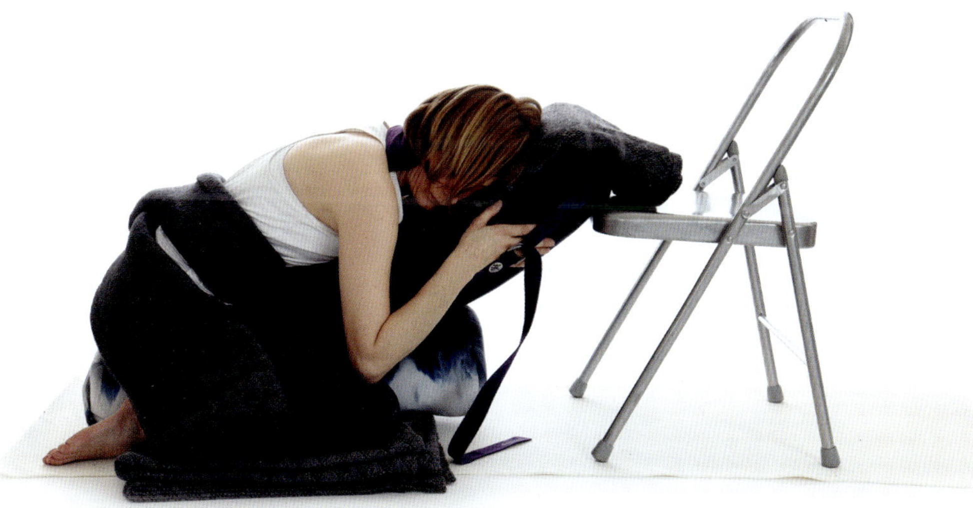

FIGURE 4.2 Audrey demonstrates Salamba Balasana seated on a round bolster to reduce pressure on the knees and make the posture more accessible and comfortable.

- Slip your fingers under the strap, resting your palms on the sides of the second bolster. Keep your forearms parallel to the top bolster, with your shoulders relaxed to avoid tension.
- Remain in the pose for 3–5 minutes, allowing your body to fully release into the support. Then gently turn your head to the opposite side to maintain balance and symmetry. Relax for another 3–5 minutes before coming out of the pose.

ALTERNATIVE SETUP WITHOUT A CHAIR

If you do not have knee issues, you can opt for a quicker setup without a chair. For this variation, you will need: 1 bolster, 3 bricks, 3 blankets, 1 strap, 1 scarf, 1 eye pillow.

- Prepare the bolster: Loop a yoga strap lengthwise around a bolster and secure it tightly. Adjust the strap so it is snug enough to support your hands during the pose.
- Place the prepared bolster lengthwise on your yoga mat, supported by two bricks: one positioned vertically under the top and the other horizontally at the middle. This setup creates a stable 45-degree angle (fig. 4.3).
- Cover the second bolster with a single-fold rectangular blanket to slightly elevate your torso and provide additional padding for comfort. Place a third brick lengthwise at the base of the setup, where you will sit.

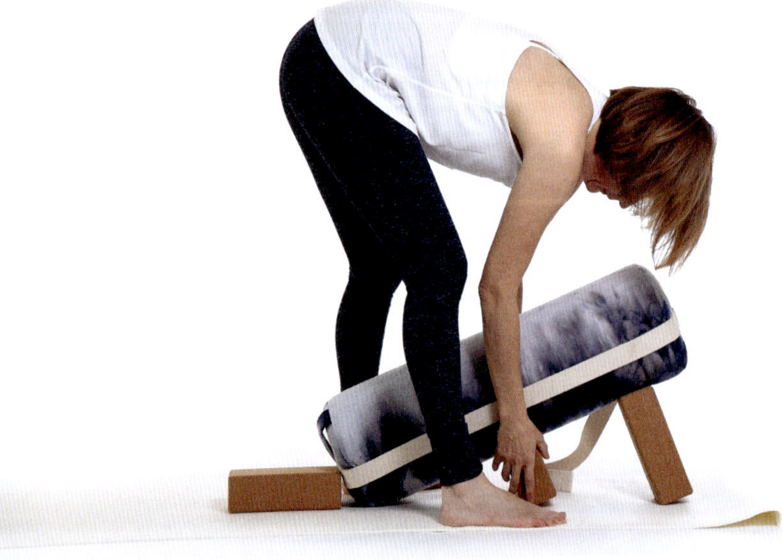

FIGURE 4.3 Audrey prepares a variation of Salamba Balasana with fewer props: a round bolster tilted at 45 degrees on two bricks, a strap to support the hands, and a third brick to elevate the pelvis.

- Sit on the brick with your knees bent and your shins resting on the mat. Keep your feet pointing straight back to ensure proper alignment and prevent unnecessary strain on the inner knees.
- If you experience any discomfort in your knees, rise up and gently draw your calf muscles toward your heels. This will create additional space for knee flexion, helping to alleviate strain on the joints. Then lower yourself to sit down.
- If necessary, place a standard blanket widthwise under your ankles for added support. Tuck the thin edge of the blanket under your ankle joints to reduce stiffness and provide comfort for your feet and ankles (fig. 4.4).
- Before leaning forward, fold a blanket lengthwise three times to create a narrow strip. Place the folded blanket horizontally across your abdomen, between your lower ribs and hip bones. Ensure it's under your abdomen, not under your hips. Take both ends of the blanket and wrap them around your pelvis, similar to tying a kimono belt. Secure it with a knot at your back, providing gentle compression to relieve menstrual discomfort.
- Lean your torso forward, resting comfortably. Turn your head to one side and slightly tuck your chin. Your back should curve outward in slight flexion from the base of your neck all the way to your pelvis. Ensure the back of your neck is long and not extended. If necessary, adjust the bolster's angle to improve alignment.

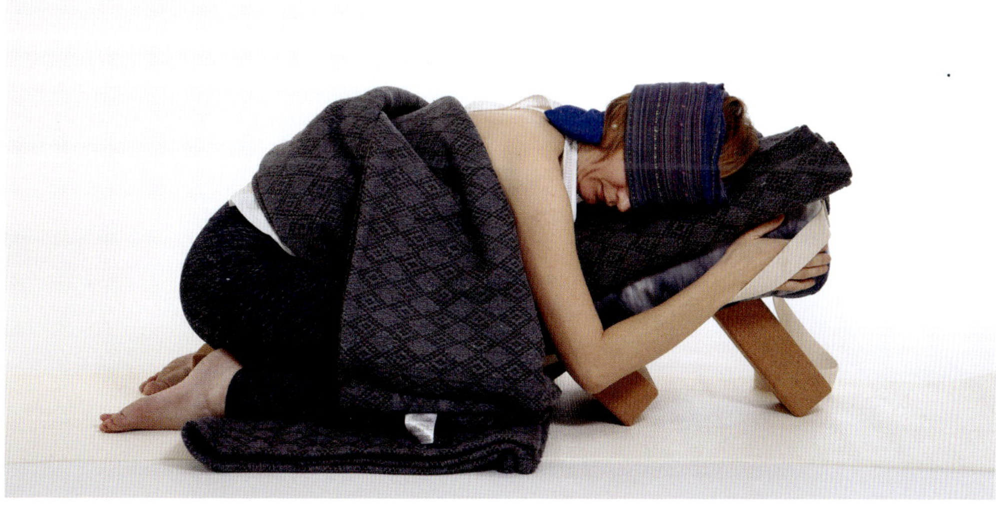

FIGURE 4.4 Audrey demonstrates a variation of Salamba Balasana, resting on a round bolster at a 45-degree angle with a blanket wrapped around the belly to encourage deep abdominal release.

- Use a scarf tucked under your face to drape over your eyes. Place an eye pillow at the back of your neck for added relaxation. Cover yourself with a blanket for warmth and comfort.
- Slip your fingers under the strap, resting your palms on the sides of the bolster. Keep your forearms parallel to the bolster, with your shoulders relaxed to avoid tension.
- Stay in the pose for 2–3 minutes, allowing your body to fully release into the support. Afterward, gently turn your head to the opposite side to maintain balance and symmetry. Remain for another 2–3 minutes before slowly coming out of the pose.

GUIDING STUDENTS THROUGH RELAXATION

During the practice, you can use the following guidance to help students relax deeply and connect with the pose:

- Slightly lower your chin toward your chest, allowing your neck to soften. Breathe naturally through your nose, letting each inhale and exhale flow with ease.
- Shift your awareness to your belly and pelvis. As you inhale, imagine that your breath fills the entire belly and pelvis. As you exhale, visualize your breath flowing out through your navel and sinking into the props below you.
- Imagine breathing in through the back of your navel and out through the front, releasing into the blanket around you.
- Take a few more deep breaths, expanding your belly and pelvis on each inhale. As you exhale, feel your belly and pelvis soften, melting into the support of the props. Let this gentle release travel up your spine.
- Imagine your breath flowing through your heart. On the inhale, imagine your breath coming in behind your shoulder blades. On the exhale, feel it flowing through your heart, down into the bolster. Inhale through the back, and exhale through the heart, surrendering deeper into the pose with each breath.
- Allow your entire spine to fully relax onto the bolster, as if you're embracing it. Let the support beneath you carry the weight of your body.
- Release all effort in your legs. Let go from the back of your hips down through the back of your thighs and all the way to your feet. Feel the sides of your waist soften, allowing tension to dissolve down the sides of your legs to your ankles.

- Let go from deep within your pelvis and abdomen, allowing relaxation to flow down the front of your thighs to your feet and from the inner groin through your inner legs to your inner ankles. Let your legs rest fully.
- As the ground holds you, allow your breath to rise and fall like gentle waves, gradually releasing all tension.

TRANSITIONING OUT OF THE POSE

- After completing the pose on both sides, bring your awareness back to the sensations of contact with the ground and the props.
- When you feel ready, release your hands from the belt and use them to help you sit up while you exhale.

Savasana (Corpse Pose) with Elevated and Weighted Ankles

20–25 MINUTES

This Savasana variation is particularly effective for relieving abdominal and lower-back pain often experienced during the menstrual cycle. By gently elevating and adding weight to the ankles, this pose helps reduce swelling in the legs, improves circulation in the pelvic region, and alleviates tension in the lower body.

I often guide this practice with a soft belly breathing technique inspired by Jillian Pransky, yoga teacher and author of *Deep Listening*. This method enhances the restorative benefits of the pose, creating a calming and supportive experience that is especially beneficial for people living with endometriosis.

CONTRAINDICATIONS

After the first trimester of pregnancy, it is recommended to practice Side-Lying Savasana on your left side (fig. 4.20).

PROPS NEEDED

1 yoga mat, 4 blankets, 1 sandbag, 2 bricks, 1 eye pillow

SETTING UP THE POSE

- Sit on your yoga mat with your knees bent and feet flat on the floor.
- Fold a standard blanket into two layers and place it horizontally at the top of your mat. The higher layer should support your head, with the thick edge placed under the C7 vertebra for optimal support, while the lower layer, with its thin edge, supports the top of your shoulder blades.
- Lay a stack of two single-fold rectangular blankets lengthwise on the floor in front of you. These blankets will support your shins and feet. Ensure that your knees rest comfortably on the edge of the blankets. Your legs should not be elevated more than 6 inches above the floor to avoid interfering with menstrual energy.
- Rotate your legs gently inward to align them in a neutral position, and place a sandbag across your ankles to anchor your legs to the blankets (fig. 4.5). This alignment can alleviate sacroiliac discomfort, while the added weight promotes grounding and relaxes the lower body.
- Cover your legs with a blanket for warmth and comfort.
- Lie on your back and position your arms at a minimum 45-degree angle from your torso. Rest the edge of each hand on a yoga brick to place your shoulder joints in a neutral, deeply relaxing position (fig. 4.6).

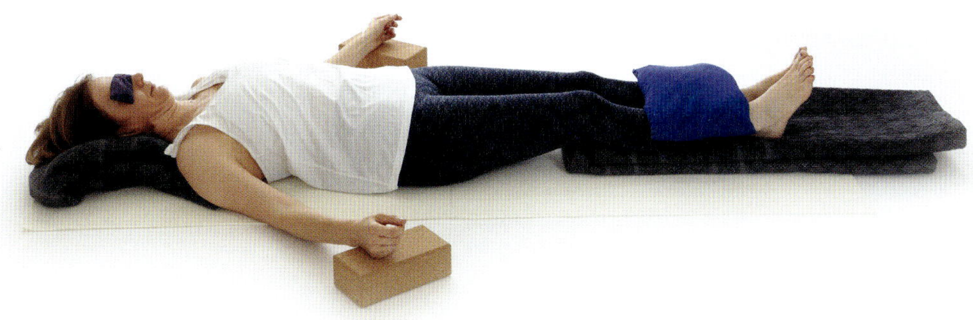

FIGURE 4.5 Audrey demonstrates Savasana with Elevated and Weighted Ankles so the shins are level with or above the abdomen, relaxing the lower back without affecting menstruation.

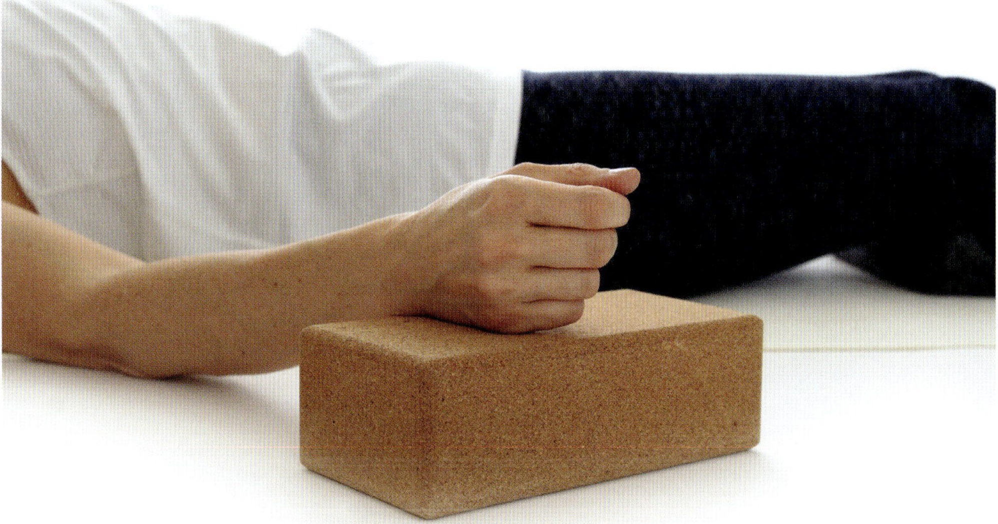

FIGURE 4.6 The wrist supported by a cork brick in Savasana, allowing the hand to relax in a neutral position and encouraging release in the shoulder girdle.

- Adjust the blanket under your head, rolling its outer edges along the sides of your neck, your head, and your outer shoulders to provide complete support.
- Cover yourself completely with a blanket to stay warm and cozy. Place a small eye pillow over your eyes to encourage deeper relaxation and reduce light exposure.
- Remain in this pose for 20–25 minutes, allowing your body to fully release and rest in silence.

GUIDING STUDENTS THROUGH RELAXATION

During the practice, you can use the following guidance to help students relax deeply and connect with the pose:

- Begin by taking deep breaths, inhaling and exhaling through the nose. When breathing through the nose, the exhale is naturally longer than the inhale. This lowers the heart rate, which in turn calms the nervous system.
- Let your body settle onto the ground and bring your awareness to your breath. With each inhale, imagine spreading softness through your belly. With each exhale, imagine your abdomen letting go of any resistance: inhale softness, exhale resistance. With each inhale, visualize your breath nurturing your belly. With each exhale, let your breath dissolve any tension.
- Allow thoughts, emotions, and sensations to rise and fall in and out of a spacious belly. Jillian Pransky used to say that our abdomen is our emotional center. When we soften it, a variety of feelings, thoughts, images, and memories may surface.[5]
- Embrace all that rises and falls. If you find yourself caught up in a thought or emotion, simply acknowledge it with compassion and shift your awareness gently back to the sensations of your breath.

TRANSITIONING OUT OF THE POSE

- At the end of the practice, place your hands gently on your belly and feel your breath move under your hands. Welcome your breath into your hands.
- At your own pace, turn your knees inward.
- Gently press your lower back into the ground and carefully slide your legs out from under the sandbag.
- Bend one knee, then the other, and slowly roll onto your side. Allow the eye pillow to fall off naturally. Rest here for at least three deep breaths.
- When you feel ready, gradually open your eyes and use your hands to support yourself as you return to a seated position.
- With your eyes still closed, take a few moments to observe the effects of the practice on your body, mind, and emotions. Notice any shifts without judgment or analysis—simply acknowledge what is present.
- Conclude your practice by setting an intention to remain connected to your breath and your belly as you move forward with your day.

Restorative Yoga Sequences for Menstruation

The following sequences are specifically designed to support you during your menstrual cycle, offering effective relief from dysmenorrhea while fostering relaxation and enhancing overall well-being.

SEQUENCE 2

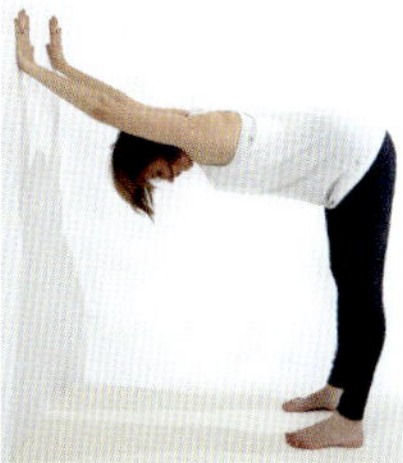

Ardha Svanasana *(page 158)*
1–2 minutes

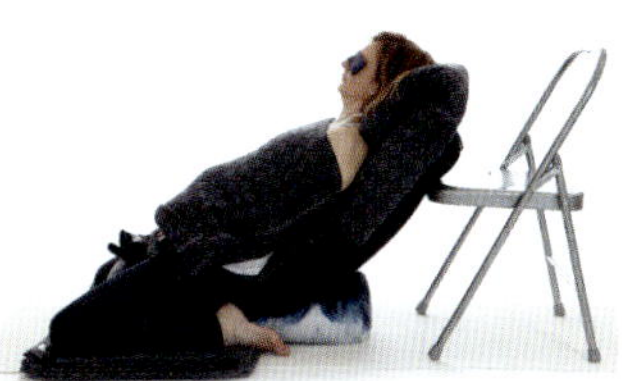

Salamba Supta Virasana *(page 161)*
20 minutes

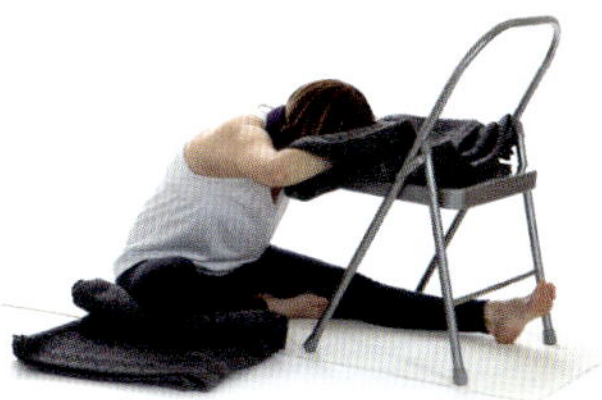

Salamba Janu Sirsasana *(page 74)*
3–5 minutes each side

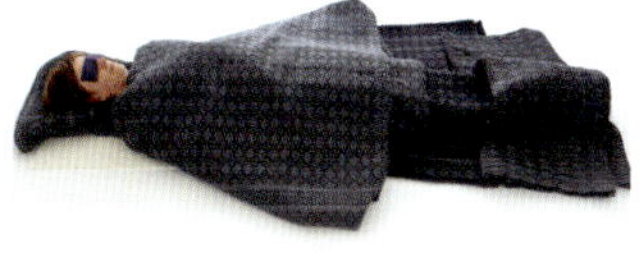

Swaddled Savasana *(page 100)*
20–25 minutes

SEQUENCE 3

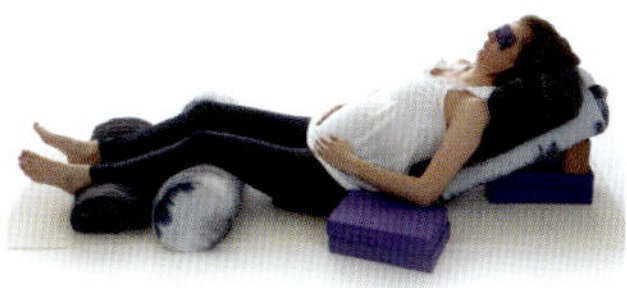

Chaise Longue Pose *(page 28)*
20 minutes

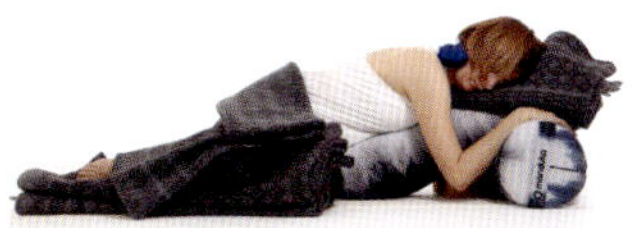

Salamba Bharadvajasana *(page 53)*
5 minutes each side

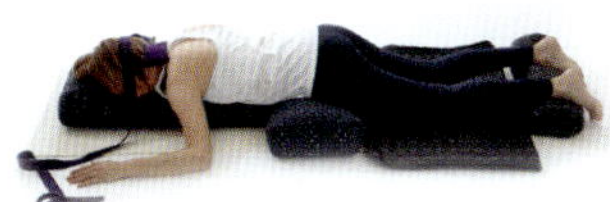

Adho Mukha Savasana with Two Bolsters (page 149)
15–20 minutes

SEQUENCE 4

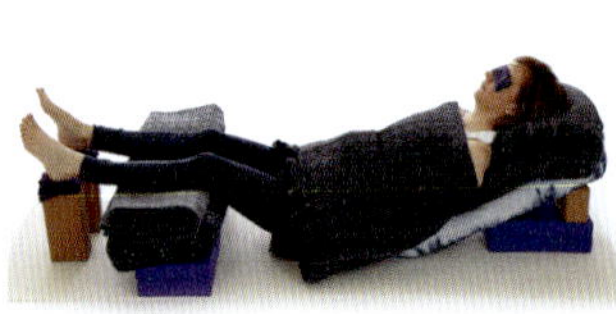

Salamba Navasana with Bent Legs (page 78)
20–25 minutes

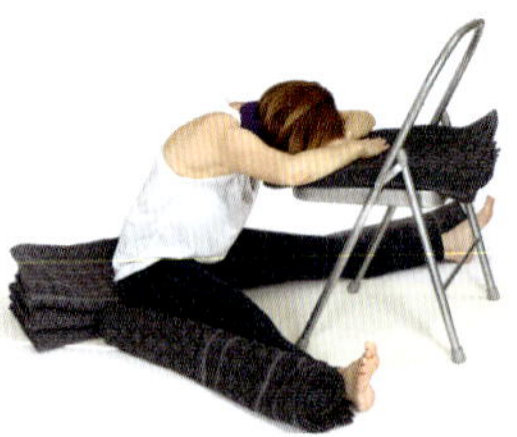

Salamba Upavistha Konasana (page 38)
5 minutes

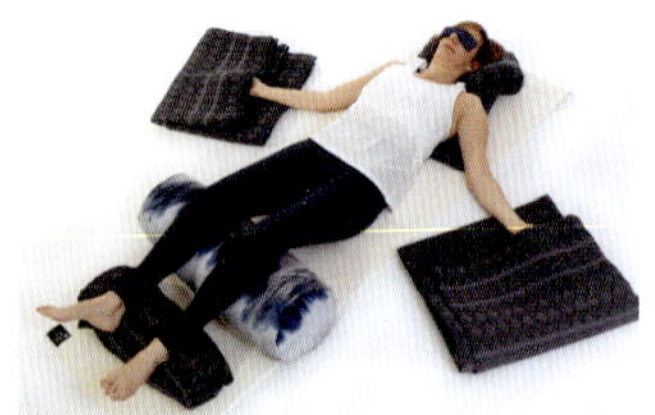

Salamba Savasana (page 41)
20 minutes

Supporting Fertility

Infertility affects approximately 15 percent of couples worldwide, with causes varying across both sexes. Notably, stress has been identified as a significant factor influencing fertility. A 2014 study led by Courtney Denning-Johnson Lynch at Ohio State University's Wexner Medical Center found that people exhibiting high levels of alpha-amylase—a stress biomarker—experienced a 29 percent reduction in monthly conception rates and were over twice as likely to meet the clinical criteria for infertility compared to those with lower levels.[6]

Practicing Restorative Yoga for approximately twenty minutes activates the parasympathetic nervous system, the body's rest-and-digest state. This activation allows energy-consuming physiological processes to slow down, enabling the body to redirect resources toward reproductive health. While specific poses offer physical benefits, the essence of Restorative Yoga lies in its capacity to induce profound relaxation and surrender, cultivating an optimal environment for healing and equilibrium.

This state of letting go is especially important when facing infertility, a journey often fraught with feelings of helplessness. Alleviating emotional strain begins with embracing the present moment, acknowledging and accepting personal and shared emotions—especially the fears and uncertainties surrounding conception—and prioritizing self-care. Restorative Yoga serves as a transformative tool in navigating these challenges, bolstering emotional resilience while gently preparing the body for pregnancy.

Certain Restorative Yoga poses also contribute to hormonal balance and menstrual cycle regulation. Although regular menstrual cycles are generally the norm, fluctuations can occur and may impact fertility. Irregular cycles can manifest in various ways, including:

- infrequent periods (oligomenorrhea)
- frequent periods (polymenorrhea)
- spotting between periods
- heavy or prolonged bleeding (menorrhagia)
- absence of menstruation for over three months (amenorrhea)

Factors contributing to irregular cycles include significant weight fluctuations, chronic stress, and medical conditions such as uterine fibroids, polycystic ovary syndrome (PCOS), and hypothyroidism. An irregular cycle not only indicates physiological imbalance but also heightens bodily vulnerability; for instance, inadequate thyroid hormone production can elevate miscarriage risk.

The Restorative Yoga sequences detailed in this chapter are specifically designed to support both fertility and hormonal regulation. By focusing on poses that stimulate the pituitary gland and enhance feminine energy, such as inversions and backbends, these practices help address infertility, irregular cycles, hypothyroidism, and endometriosis. Beyond their physical benefits, these sequences promote stress reduction and cultivate a mind-set of detachment, fostering emotional resilience and overall well-being.

Salamba Sarvangasana (Supported Shoulderstand) with a Chair

5–10 MINUTES

Sarvangasana, commonly known as the shoulderstand, is among the most beneficial asanas due to its profound and comprehensive impact on the body. It positively influences the abdominal organs, heart, lungs, thyroid gland, and nervous system. Its therapeutic benefits extend to alleviating menstrual disorders, stimulating fertility, and fostering overall physical and emotional balance.

In her seminal book, *Yoga: A Gem for Women*, Geeta Iyengar refers to Sarvangasana as the "mother of asanas." She writes, "As a mother strives throughout her life to ensure her children's happiness, the mother of asanas endeavors to establish peace and health in the body."[7] This poetic analogy highlights the nurturing and restorative qualities of the pose. Sarvangasana's influence on the nervous system fosters patience and emotional balance—qualities that are particularly essential for navigating the challenges associated with fertility and hormonal imbalances.

One of the key physiological mechanisms of Sarvangasana lies in the position of the chin, which forms Jalandhara Bandha (Chin Lock). This subtle adjustment enhances blood flow to the thyroid and parathyroid glands, optimizing their function and supporting the body's physical and mental equilibrium. Additionally, the gentle pressure applied to the baroreceptors in the carotid sinuses can help lower heart rate and blood pressure, fostering a state of homeostasis. These effects make Sarvangasana especially effective in soothing the mind, calming the nervous system, and alleviating stress.

Beyond its hormonal and nervous system benefits, Sarvangasana is highly therapeutic for respiratory conditions such as asthma, bronchitis, and sore throats. It also supports digestion, elimination, and detoxification while improving blood circulation, making it an excellent remedy for chronic fatigue and sluggish metabolism.

PRACTICE GUIDELINES

- Perform the following three poses in succession without exiting the sequence:
  1. Salamba Sarvangasana
  2. Salamba Urdhva Dhanurasana
  3. Viparita Baddha Konasana
- Practice under the guidance of a qualified yoga teacher if you are unfamiliar with these poses.
- New practitioners should opt for more accessible poses, such as Supta Baddha Konasana (fig. 4.1), Viparita Baddha Konasana (fig. 4.10), and Adho Mukha Savasana (fig. 4.16).

CONTRAINDICATIONS

- pregnancy
- menstruation
- indigestion
- herniated disc
- whiplash
- pinched nerve
- chronic neck pain or injuries
- sinusitis or colds
- gastroesophageal reflux disease (GERD)
- spondylolysis and spondylolisthesis
- high blood pressure
- retinal detachment
- glaucoma

PROPS NEEDED

2 yoga mats, 1 yoga chair, 1 bolster, 7–8 blankets, bricks or blocks, 1 eye pillow

SETTING UP THE POSE

Position the Chair

- Place a yoga chair on your yoga mat approximately 18 inches from a wall. This wall will serve as support for your feet during the pose. Note that the wall is not shown in the images.

Prepare the Seat

- Drape a standard-fold blanket across the backrest of the chair to soften the contact with your legs.
- Place a single-fold square blanket over the seat of the chair, letting it hang slightly over the front edge.
- To prevent the blanket from sliding as you move into the pose, you may fold a sticky yoga mat and place it under the blanket for added grip.

Set Shoulder Support

- Arrange a combination of a bolster and double-fold blankets in front of the chair to provide support for your shoulders.

Prepare Head Support

- In front of the bolster, perpendicular to it, place 2–3 double-fold blankets to support your head.
- Adjust the number of blankets so your head rests at an incline of approximately 45 degrees, with your chin slightly elevated. Your weight should rest on the top of your shoulders.
- Take time to experiment with the height and arrangement of bolsters and blankets to achieve optimal support and alignment.

Set Foot Support

- Arrange a combination of yoga blocks or bricks of equal height on the floor, positioning them on either side of the back legs of the chair. These blocks will serve as a secure platform to support your feet while practicing Salamba Urdhva Dhanurasana.
- Double-check that the blocks are stable and properly aligned to provide comfortable and reliable support for your feet throughout the pose.

GETTING INTO THE POSE

- Sit astride the chair, facing the backrest, and hold onto it with both hands for stability.
- One leg at a time, swing your legs over the backrest, keeping them bent to gently squeeze the chair. Move your body as close to the backrest as possible (fig. 4.7).

LOWERING INTO THE POSE

- Hold the sides of the chair firmly with your hands and lean back slowly, sliding slightly toward the front edge of the seat.
- Carefully lower your back, arching over the seat's front edge, until your shoulders rest on the bolster and your head is supported by the blankets on the floor. Avoid tensing or contracting your neck.

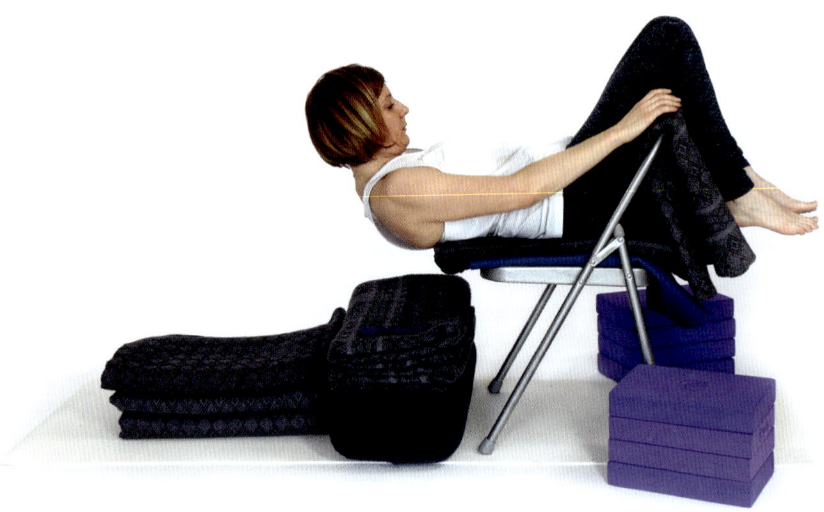

FIGURE 4.7 Audrey prepares Salamba Sarvangasana by bringing her pelvis close to the backrest and squeezing the chair with her legs before gently lowering into position.

ALIGN YOUR HEAD AND TORSO

- Position your head so it rests on the blankets just beneath the external occipital protuberance (the base of the skull).
- Ensure your sacrum rests fully on the seat, while the lower ribs lightly touch the blanket on the front edge of the chair.
- Check that the C7 vertebra (the bony prominence at the base of your neck) is supported by the bolster and blankets, allowing your neck to relax completely. When you touch the back of your neck, the nuchal ligament should not feel taut or protruding.

GRIP THE CHAIR FOR STABILITY

- Without moving your torso, slip your hands, one at a time, between the chair legs to grasp the back legs. Your palms should face each other.
- If reaching the back legs is difficult, use a yoga strap looped around the back legs for assistance.
- Once securely holding the legs, roll your shoulders under your body one at a time, standing firmly on your collarbones rather than pressing into your shoulders. Lift your mid-thoracic spine to open your chest.

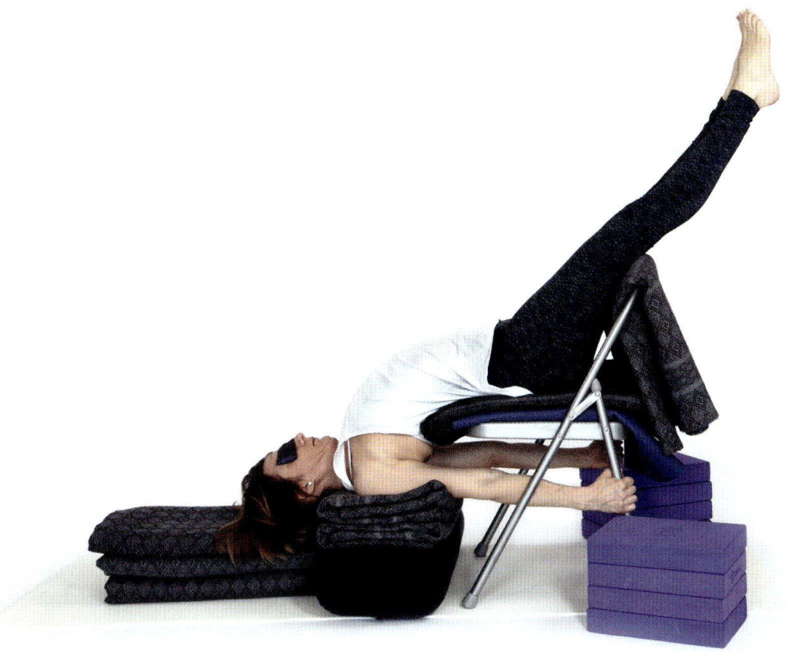

FIGURE 4.8 Audrey demonstrates Salamba Sarvangasana with the head lower than the shoulders, supported by blankets, pelvis on a chair, legs extended upward. The feet can rest on a wall (not shown).

POSITION YOUR LEGS

- On an exhale, straighten your legs and rest your feet on the wall, allowing the backrest of the chair to support your legs.
- Press your tailbone firmly into the seat to stimulate and open the abdominal region (fig. 4.8).

FINAL ADJUSTMENTS

- Cover yourself with a blanket to stay warm, and place an eye pillow gently over your eyes to promote relaxation.

DURATION

- Maintain this supported Sarvangasana for 5–10 minutes or longer, as your comfort and practice allow.
- Breathe naturally through your nose, allowing your body to rest deeply in the pose.

IF YOU EXPERIENCE DISCOMFORT IN THE NECK

- Come out of the pose. Neck discomfort often indicates inadequate support under your shoulders or an excessive elevation under your head.
- Relax and take a moment to assess the arrangement of your props. Adjust the height of the blankets under your head and shoulders to ensure proper alignment and support. A balanced setup is key to maintaining comfort and avoiding strain.
- Once you have adjusted your props, carefully reenter the pose, paying close attention to your alignment and ensuring your neck feels relaxed and supported.
- If discomfort persists despite adjustments, transition directly to Viparita Baddha Konasana, a restorative alternative that provides many of the same benefits without strain on the neck.

GUIDING STUDENTS THROUGH RELAXATION

During the practice, you can use the following guidance to help students relax deeply and connect with the pose:

- Bring your awareness to your body. Notice all the places where your body connects with the props supporting you. Take several deep breaths and progressively release all your body weight down toward the ground. Trust the props to hold you completely.
- Release any tension in your legs and pelvis. Let go of any gripping or holding.
- Invite ease into your head, neck, and shoulders. Feel these areas soften as you settle further into stillness.
- Now visualize a revitalizing stream of water. Imagine it flowing in through the soles of your feet, traveling down through your legs, and pooling gently in your belly. Feel it streaming into your heart, cleansing the chest, and moving downward through the throat. Finally, it flows out through the crown of your head, washing away any tension and leaving a sense of clarity and renewal in its path.
- Let your breath move like waves. With each rise and fall, feel yourself softening more deeply.
- Embrace the quietness within. With each exhale, feel your mind grow calmer as a serene stillness settles in, leaving you refreshed and at peace.

Salamba Urdhva Dhanurasana (Supported Upward Bow Pose)

5 MINUTES

This supported variation of Urdhva Dhanurasana offers numerous benefits. By gently stretching and opening the pelvic region, this pose enhances the health and vitality of the pelvic organs, supporting reproductive and hormonal balance. The pose also encourages the upward flow of apana energy, which is associated with grounding, elimination, and the release of physical and emotional tension.

In addition to its physical benefits, Salamba Urdhva Dhanurasana fosters a sense of spaciousness in the front of the body, allowing for deep, restorative breathing. This openness helps calm the mind, soothe the nervous system, and promote a state of relaxation and inner balance. It is an excellent pose for relieving fatigue, releasing stress, and cultivating a sense of emotional harmony.

CONTRAINDICATIONS

- pregnancy
- menstruation
- indigestion
- herniated disc
- whiplash
- pinched nerve
- chronic neck pain or injuries
- sinusitis or colds
- gastroesophageal reflux disease (GERD)
- spondylolysis and spondylolisthesis
- high blood pressure
- retinal detachment
- glaucoma

TRANSITIONING TO SALAMBA URDHVA DHANURASANA

- From Salamba Sarvangasana, gently bend one knee and place that foot onto the backrest of the chair for support. Repeat with the other leg, bringing both feet to rest on the chair's backrest.
- Carefully lower one foot at a time onto the corresponding blocks, ensuring the blocks are positioned securely and at a height that allows your feet to comfortably reach them.

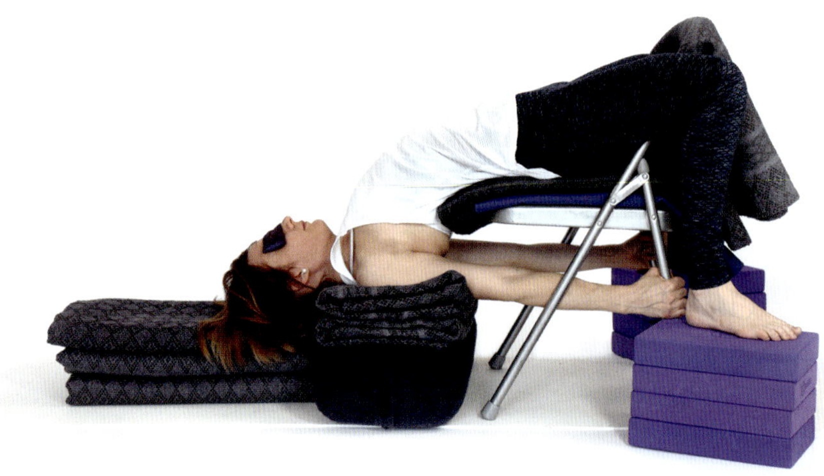

FIGURE 4.9 Audrey demonstrates a variation of Salamba Urdhva Dhanurasana with the pelvis resting on a chair and feet on blocks to open and stimulate the abdominal organs.

- Press your feet firmly into the blocks, keeping them slightly turned outward. This outward rotation helps create space in the hips.
- Engage your leg muscles to maintain stability and support.
- Focus on lengthening the area from your diaphragm down to your feet, creating a gentle stretch along the front of your body (fig. 4.9).
- Allow your abdomen to soften as you breathe deeply, promoting relaxation and release.
- Stay in this supported variation for a few minutes, breathing naturally and focusing on the expansive sensation in your body. Let the pose gently open your hips, abdomen, and chest while calming your mind.

GUIDING STUDENTS THROUGH RELAXATION

During the practice, you can use the following guidance to help students relax deeply and connect with the pose:

- Allow your body to settle fully into the props, letting them provide all the support you need. Breathe deeply into the present moment, and with each exhale, release any tension you're holding.
- Let go of any need to control the pose and instead invite the pose to naturally work its magic on your abdomen. Your belly is open, nourished by the grounding apana energy.

- Feel your abdomen rise and fall with each breath, like the ebb and flow of the sea. In this nurturing position, all your abdominal organs are revitalized and refreshed.
- The relaxation extends gently to your back. Sense each vertebra beginning to release as this wave of ease travels up your spine.
- As you rest here, welcome this growing sense of calm and well-being within you.

TRANSITIONING TO THE NEXT POSE

- Gently take off the eye pillow and set it aside to prepare for movement.
- As you exhale, bend one knee and place your foot carefully onto the backrest of the chair. Repeat with the other leg, ensuring both feet are securely positioned for support.
- Let go of your grip on the chair legs and gradually begin to slide your body downward off the chair, allowing your pelvis to gently rest on the bolster. Ensure your shoulders and head are supported comfortably by the blankets arranged on the floor.
- Carefully push the chair slightly toward the end of the mat to create more space for your legs.
- Once adjusted, rest your lower legs comfortably on the seat of the chair, allowing your knees to bend naturally.

Viparita Baddha Konasana (Inverted Bound Angle Pose)

5–10 MINUTES

Viparita Baddha Konasana is a Restorative Yoga pose that combines the benefits of Baddha Konasana (Bound Angle Pose) with a gentle inversion. This asana promotes deep relaxation and provides several therapeutic benefits:

- **hip opener**: By allowing the knees to fall outward, this pose effectively opens the hips.
- **enhanced blood circulation**: The gentle inversion promotes increased blood flow to the pelvic region, including the ovaries and uterus. Improved circulation ensures that these organs receive an adequate supply of hormones and nutrients, thereby supporting their optimal functioning.
- **nervous system relaxation**: The supported inversion encourages the body to enter a state of deep relaxation, calming the nervous system and reducing stress levels.

CONTRAINDICATIONS

- pregnancy
- menstruation
- sinusitis or cold
- gastroesophageal reflux
- spondylolysis and spondylolisthesis
- retinal detachment
- glaucoma
- hiatal hernia

SETTING UP THE POSE

- From the previous pose, remove the blankets from the bolster and the floor, keeping only one under your torso.
- Use the remaining blankets to support your forearms, ensuring comfort and warmth.
- Rest your pelvis and lower ribs on the bolster, while your shoulders and head are supported by the blanket.
- Ensure that the lower ribs in your back are well supported by the bolster, creating a gentle backbend. This slight backbend stimulates the abdominal organs, particularly the lower ones.

- Your pubic bone should be level with or slightly lower than your navel. The gentle opening in the front of the pelvis encourages increased blood flow to the reproductive organs, providing them with oxygen and nutrients to support optimal function.
- Choose the arm position that feels most comfortable for you:
    - Extend your arms overhead (fig. 4.10) to release tension in the trapezius and deltoid muscles.
    - Position your arms alongside your body, as in Ardha Viparita Karani (fig. 3.3).
- Hook your feet on either side of the chair's back, allowing your knees to hang down freely.
- If your chair doesn't allow for this position, bring the soles of your feet together and let your knees fall outward into the Baddha Konasana position. If needed, you can wrap a blanket around your feet to help keep them in place.
- Cover yourself with a blanket for warmth and comfort.
- Place an eye pillow gently over your eyes to promote relaxation.
- Remain in this pose for 5–10 minutes, or longer if it feels restorative.

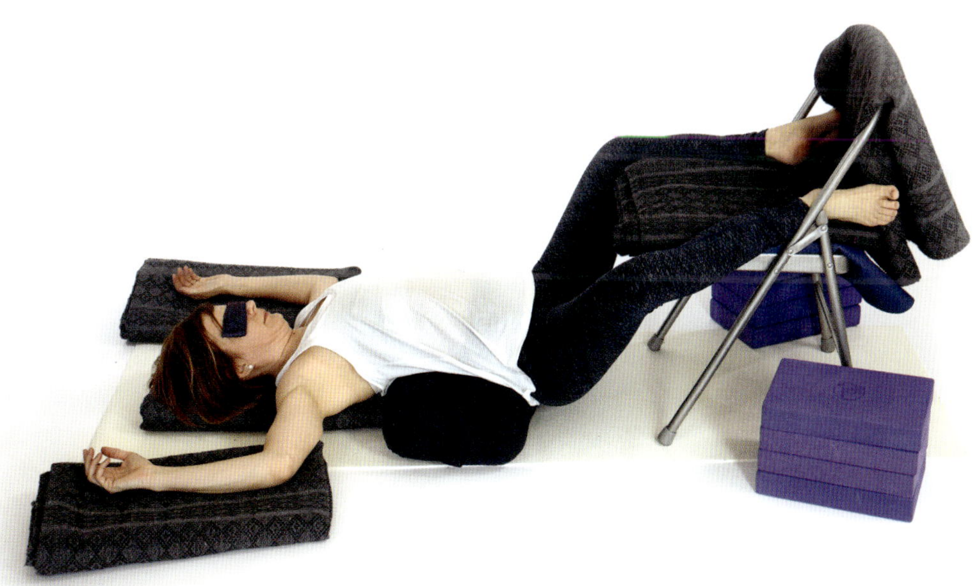

FIGURE 4.10 Audrey demonstrates Viparita Baddha Konasana with her pelvis and lower ribs supported by a bolster and the tailbone gently releasing downward.

GUIDING STUDENTS THROUGH RELAXATION

During the practice, you can use the following guidance to help students relax deeply and connect with the pose:

- Bring your awareness to your body. Begin by noticing your ankles resting on the frame of the chair. With each exhale, progressively release any effort to hold you up. Allow your knees to hang freely on either side of the chair and feel your thighs grow heavier and more at ease.
- Let your pelvis and lower back settle into the bolster. If you notice any lingering tension, imagine it dissolving and drifting away with each breath.
- Feel the relaxation spreading through your chest, thorax, and diaphragm. As you inhale, sense your breath gently expanding and opening your upper chest. With every exhale, feel your back spreading more widely across the props, melting into their support. Imagine you could breathe through the front of your chest: air entering gently through the front of the heart, and on the exhale, flowing out through the back of the heart into the ground.
- Allow your breath to release tension and soften everything it comes into contact with. As your upper back broadens, feel your neck relaxing and your throat opening. Let the nape and back of your head rest fully into the cradle of the blanket, along with your arms and hands, which feel completely supported.
- Your body becomes a revitalizing wave, flowing effortlessly with the rhythm of your breath, restoring and renewing itself with each rise and fall.

TRANSITIONING OUT OF THE POSE

- When it is time to come out of the pose, bring your awareness back to the sensations of contact with the floor and the props.
- Slowly remove the eye bag and allow your eyes to open softly, adjusting gradually to the light.
- At your own pace, slide yourself backward toward your head until your entire back is resting on the floor.
- Bend your knees and remain in this position for a few moments.
- When you feel ready, roll onto your side and return to a seated position, using your hands for support.

Ardha Halasana (Half Plow Pose)

5–10 MINUTES

Ardha Halasana is a deeply restorative pose that offers numerous physical and psychological benefits. Its therapeutic effects make it particularly valuable for overall well-being and hormonal balance.

PHYSICAL BENEFITS

- **regulating the menstrual cycle**: This pose supports hormonal balance by helping to regulate the menstrual cycle and moderate menstrual flow.
- **muscle relaxation**: It gently stretches and relaxes the back muscles, alleviating tension and reducing fatigue.
- **calming the nervous system**: The pose encourages relaxation by calming the nervous system, which can reduce stress and anxiety.
- **improved circulation**: By stimulating blood flow in the chest area, this pose enhances healthy circulation and cardiovascular function.
- **therapeutic applications**:
    - reduces the intensity of hot flashes, making it especially beneficial during menopause
    - supports kidney health by stimulating proper kidney function and improving detoxification processes

PSYCHOLOGICAL BENEFITS

- **emotional resilience**: Practicing Ardha Halasana helps cultivate psychological qualities such as self-confidence and willpower.
- **mental stability**: The calming nature of the pose fosters a sense of inner stability and balance, encouraging mental clarity and focus.

This asana harmonizes the body and mind, offering a holistic approach to health and well-being. It is particularly suitable for practitioners navigating infertility who are seeking to relieve stress while addressing physical discomforts associated with hormonal fluctuations and fatigue.

CONTRAINDICATIONS

- pregnancy
- menstruation
- during digestion

- chronic neck pain or injuries
- sinusitis or cold
- gastroesophageal reflux
- spondylolysis and spondylolisthesis
- high blood pressure
- retinal detachment
- glaucoma

PROPS NEEDED

3 yoga mats, 1 bolster, 4 blocks, 2 bricks, 8–9 blankets, 1 eye pillow

SETTING UP THE POSE

Prepare the Props

- Begin by placing your yoga mat with its short end against the wall to create a stable base for your setup.
- Position a bolster horizontally a few inches from the wall, ensuring it is parallel to the wall and aligned with the mat.
- In front of the bolster, arrange two yoga blocks on the floor side by side. Stack two additional blocks directly on top of these to create an elevated platform for shoulder support.
- Place a double-fold blanket on top of the stacked blocks to provide a soft, comfortable surface for your shoulders.
- Lay a folded nonslip yoga mat over the blanket to prevent slipping as you enter and hold the pose.
- Confirm that all props are aligned, secure, and evenly stacked to maintain stability and prevent movement during the pose.

Achieve the Correct Elevation

- Ensure the height of your stacked blocks and props elevates your shoulders by 6–8 inches above the level of your occiput (the back of your head).
- Proper elevation is crucial to provide shoulder support and keep your neck free of tension. Your throat should feel open and unrestricted.

Set Up the Chair

- Position a chair above the area where your head will rest, ensuring it is aligned with your body's setup.
- Place a single-fold square blanket under the chair to support your head.
- Stack several single-fold square blankets on the seat of the chair, adjusting their height so they reach the top of your thighs when in position. Ensure the blankets are evenly placed to keep your feet level with your hip joints.
- To prevent the blankets from sliding as you move into the pose, you may fold a sticky yoga mat and place it under the blankets for added grip.

ENTER THE POSE

- Sit on your heels at one end of the bolster, facing the center of the room.
- If the bolster is on your right, lean forward, bringing your chest toward your thighs, and slip your right arm across your chest.
- Inhale, and as you exhale, roll over onto your back, simultaneously swinging your legs up the wall. Position your head under the chair, with your shoulders on the blocks.
- Ensure the tops of your shoulders are positioned 3–4 inches away from the edge of the blocks. This spacing provides the necessary room to roll gradually onto the tops of your shoulders while maintaining stability. Proper alignment prevents your shoulders from sliding off the blocks and avoids placing undue pressure on your neck, ensuring a safe and supportive pose.
- Place your feet on the wall, about 10–12 inches apart.
- Inhale, and as you exhale, engage your abdominal muscles to curl up gradually. Avoid pushing with your legs to keep your shoulders securely on the blocks.
- Your lower legs should be perpendicular to the wall, and your knees bent at a 90-degree angle.

Position Your Hands and Legs

- Interlock your hands behind your back, straighten your elbows, and press your arms downward to lift your torso.

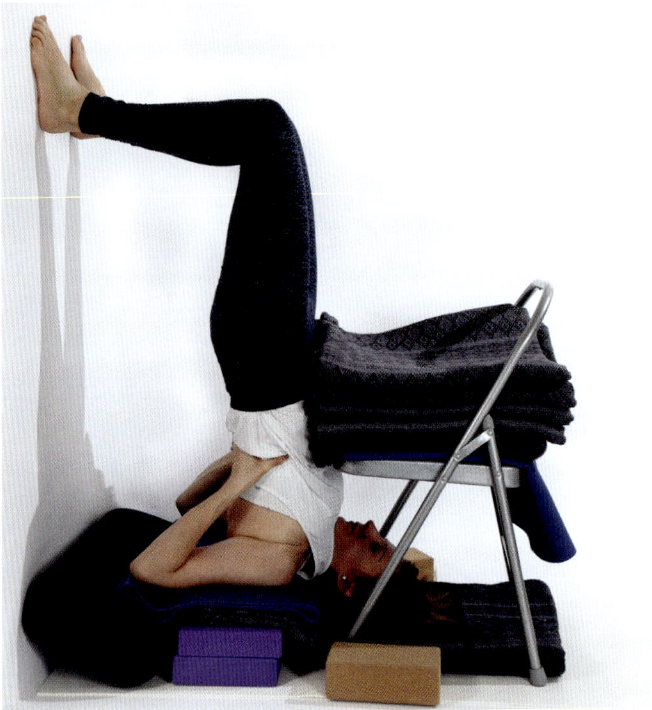

FIGURE 4.11 Audrey demonstrates how to enter Ardha Halasana by performing a shoulderstand with the feet pressing into the wall and the shoulders elevated to reduce pressure on the neck.

- Externally rotate your upper arms, tucking the outer edges slightly under your body one at a time by gently rocking side to side.
- Place your hands on your back with your thumbs pointing toward the front of your body and your fingers parallel to your ribs.
- Gradually move your hands down along your back until they rest under your lower ribs. Use your hands to push your lower ribs forward, and lift your sternum (fig. 4.11).

Adjust Your Alignment

- Ensure your sternum is vertical, your throat is relaxed, and your neck feels free. If you touch the back of your neck, the nuchal ligament should not feel taut or protruding.
- If this alignment isn't achieved, exit the pose gently and add an additional double-fold blanket under your shoulders for better support.

TRANSITION TO SALAMBA SARVANGASANA

- Lift your legs one at a time through the balls of the feet, internally rotate your thighs, and keep your legs straight.
- Stay here for a few breaths or more.

TRANSITION TO ARDHA HALASANA

- On an exhale, bend one knee and place one thigh, then the other, onto the seat of the chair.
- Slide your legs onto the chair seat one at a time, ensuring the top edges of your thighs rest securely on the blankets on the chair.
- Move your legs as far through the chair as possible, so the very top of your thighs rests on the seat.
- Rotate your thighs outward, allowing the inner quadriceps to rest directly on the blankets for added comfort.

ENSURE PROPER ALIGNMENT

- Check that your hip joints are positioned slightly in front of your shoulders, allowing your upper body to hang from the chair.
- There should be no tension in your shoulders, neck, and throat; if tension persists, add an extra blanket to the chair for better support.
- Like in Salamba Sarvangasana with a Chair, it may take several adjustments to find the right combination of props to suit your body. Be patient: Achieving the correct setup leads to maximum comfort and relaxation.

FINAL ADJUSTMENTS

- Place your arms at the sides of your head.
- For added comfort, rest your forearms on yoga bricks.
- Ask someone to place a sandbag on the back of your thighs for grounding, and cover yourself with a blanket for warmth.
- Place an eye pillow over your eyes to promote deeper relaxation.
- Stay in the pose for 5–10 minutes or longer, breathing naturally through your nose (fig. 4.12).

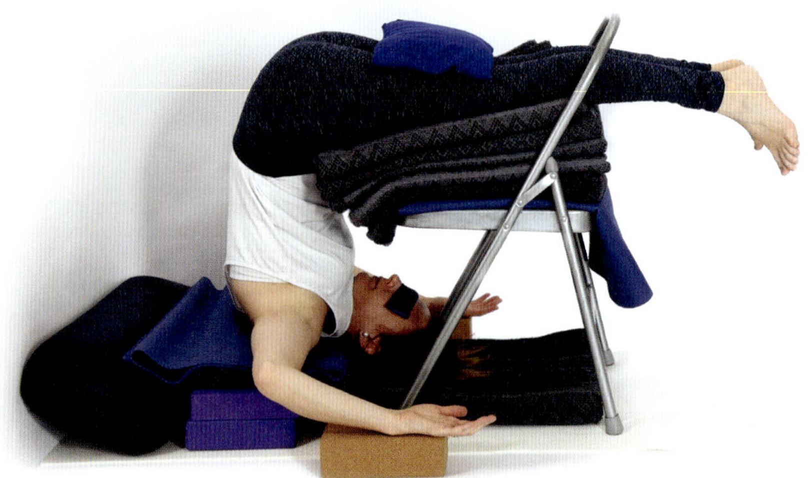

FIGURE 4.12 Audrey demonstrates Ardha Halasana with the pelvis supported by blankets on a chair and the legs extended behind, encouraging grounding and spinal release.

GUIDING STUDENTS THROUGH RELAXATION

During the practice, you can use the following guidance to help students relax deeply and connect with the pose:

- Focus your attention on your eyes. Allow them to soften and relax completely. Visualize them gently moving inward, descending toward your heart. Feel how your outer vision gradually transforms into inner sight: your insight. Let your ears follow this inward journey, noticing how your outer hearing shifts into a deep, internal listening.
- Tune in to each part of your body. Observe where tension lingers, noticing any areas of gripping or holding. Your body no longer needs to work—let the chair fully support you. With each breath, feel your body becoming lighter, softer, and more at ease.
- Use this time to connect with your deepest self. The inner movement of awareness guides you toward your essence, where you can begin to hear its soft, steady voice.
- Allow yourself to drift beyond time and space, sinking deeply into the infinite, boundless depths of your being.

TRANSITIONING OUT OF THE POSE

- Begin by taking slow, deep breaths to ground yourself and reconnect with your external surroundings.
- Gradually bring movement back into your body by wiggling your toes, then gently moving your ankles and calves.
- When you feel ready, slowly remove your eye pillow and gently open your eyes. If you have a sandbag on your thighs, ask someone to gently lift it off.
- Reach up to hold the blankets above the chair seat with your hands to maintain stability. One at a time, carefully release your legs from the back of the chair.
- Place your hands under the back of your ribs for support, with your elbows resting on the bolster. As you exhale, bend your knees and place your feet, one at a time, against the wall for stability (fig. 4.13). Slowly and with control, lower your pelvis onto the bolster (fig. 4.14).
- Once your pelvis is fully supported, take a moment to rest in this position.

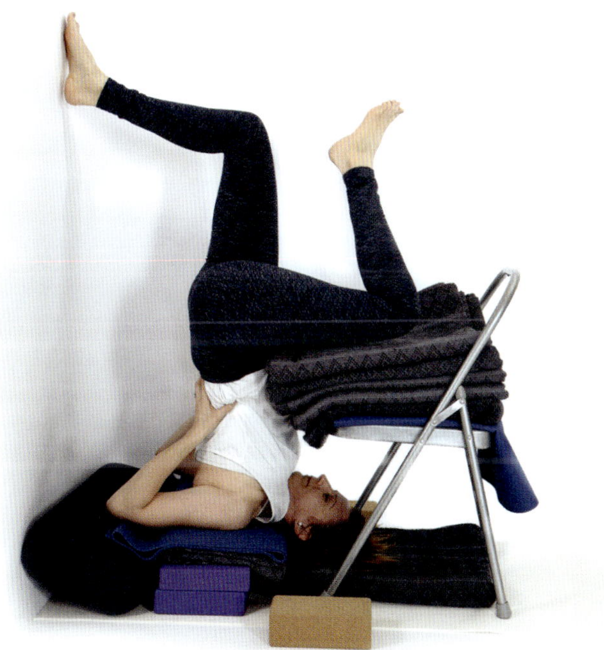

FIGURE 4.13 Audrey demonstrates how to exit Ardha Halasana by placing one foot at a time against the wall, returning to a shoulderstand with the feet supported.

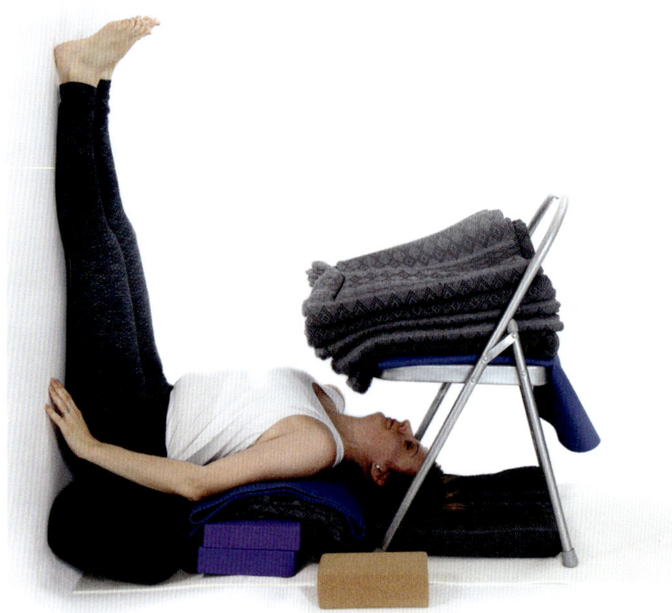

FIGURE 4.14 Audrey demonstrates the second step of exiting Ardha Halasana by resting her pelvis on the bolster, legs extended up the wall, before rolling to the side to sit up.

- At your own pace, turn onto your side, curling your legs gently toward your chest in a fetal position. Stay on your side for a few moments, breathing naturally and allowing your body to recalibrate.
- When you feel ready, use your hands to gently press yourself up into a seated position. Move slowly and mindfully, maintaining the sense of relaxation you cultivated in the pose.

Adho Mukha Savasana (Downward-Facing Relaxation Pose)

10–15 MINUTES

I have chosen to conclude this sequence with a deeply grounding pose that fosters a profound sense of safety, connection, and support from the earth. This pose invites us to release tension, both physically and emotionally, while nurturing a sense of trust and confidence in the future. Its restorative qualities make it particularly effective for relaxing the back, easing fatigue, and calming the nervous system.

CONTRAINDICATION

If you are pregnant, replace this pose with Side-Lying Savasana on your left side for optimal comfort and safety (fig. 4.20).

PROPS NEEDED

1 yoga mat, 2 bolsters, 4 blankets, 1 yoga strap, 1 eye pillow. If you don't have two bolsters, use the version with a single bolster (fig. 4.16).

SETTING UP THE POSE

- Place a bolster lengthwise at the top of your mat. Lay a second bolster perpendicularly to it, directly below the first, forming an inverted T shape. In front of the second bolster, place a standard blanket for your knees and a rolled blanket to support your ankles.
- Lie face down on your belly, turning your head to one side—whichever feels more comfortable. Rest the horizontal bolster under your upper thighs and abdomen, while the vertical bolster supports your chest and head.
- Check the curve of your lower back (lumbar lordosis). If the curve feels overly pronounced, shift slightly toward your feet to reduce the support under your thighs.
- Position the rolled blanket under your ankles. To align your hips and sacrum, momentarily lift your knees and internally rotate your thighs, letting your big toes face each other. This alignment releases tension in the sacrum, glutes, and piriformis muscles.
- Relax your arms by moving your elbows and hands slightly away from your body to release tension in the shoulders.
- Place a yoga strap over your head, allowing it to block light and support turning your head to the opposite side halfway through the pose without needing further adjustment (fig. 4.15).

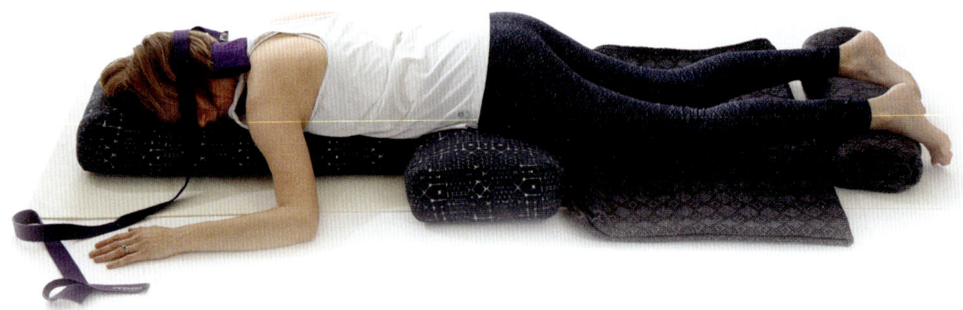

FIGURE 4.15 Audrey demonstrates Adho Mukha Savasana with the torso supported by two bolsters in a T shape, arms wide to relax the shoulders, and legs in gentle internal rotation.

- Rest an eye pillow at the back of your neck to encourage relaxation in the cervical spine.
- Close your eyes and allow your body to settle into the pose. Rest here for 10–15 minutes, fully supported by the props.

Modifications for Neck or Shoulder Tension, Cervical Herniation, or Neck Injuries

- Avoid turning your head side to side, as this may put undue pressure on the cervical discs.
- Use a single bolster positioned to support both your thighs and your torso.
- Rest your forehead on a rolled blanket to maintain a neutral cervical spine (fig. 4.16).
- This modification ensures greater comfort and minimizes strain on your neck and shoulders.

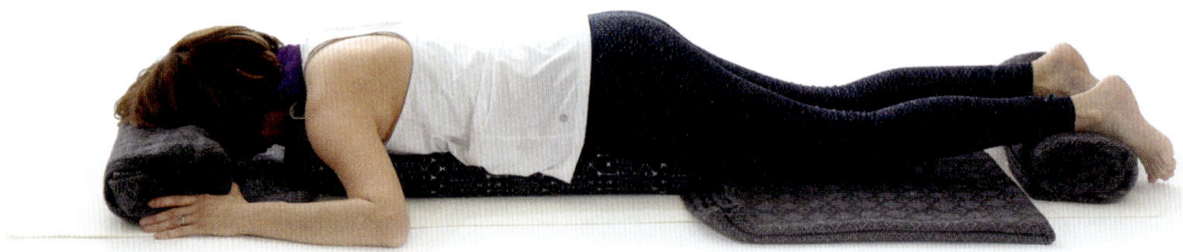

FIGURE 4.16 Audrey demonstrates a variation of Adho Mukha Savasana with the torso supported by one bolster and a rolled blanket under the forehead to ease tension in the neck.

GUIDING STUDENTS THROUGH RELAXATION

During the practice, you can use the following guidance to help students relax deeply and connect with the pose:

- Bring your attention to the back of your neck. Feel the gentle weight of the eye pillow melting away tension, slowly softening this area.
- Gently scan your body, allowing yourself to settle more fully onto the props.
- Start with your belly. As you inhale, invite a wave of relaxation into your pelvis, abdomen, and lower back. With every exhale, let your pelvis and belly soften into the props, releasing tension all the way up your spine.
- Allow your spine to relax completely, surrendering to the support of the earth and the props.
- Let go of any effort in your legs. Feel your muscles softening from your hips down to your feet. Soften any rigidity along the sides of your waist, letting it flow down your legs to your ankles. Gently release from deep within your pelvis and abdomen, down the front of your thighs, all the way to your feet. Let your legs rest in complete ease.
- Allow the earth to fully support you, creating space for your breath to flow freely. Bring your attention to the skin on your back, noticing how it moves gently with each breath. Feel the breath softly rippling along your spine, soothing and releasing tension.
- Let your breath rise and fall effortlessly. With each cycle, sense it softening your inner being and dissolving any lingering tightness.
- As you rest here, let every exhale guide you deeper into a state of peace.

TRANSITIONING OUT OF THE POSE

- Reconnect with the sensations of contact of your body with the props and the ground.
- When you feel ready, slowly slide your hands underneath your shoulders. Gather your belly into your back. Slowly come to all fours over your bolster before returning to a seated position.
- With your eyes still closed, take a few moments to observe the effects of this sequence on your body, mind, and emotions. Acknowledge any changes without judgment.

Restorative Yoga Sequences to Support Fertility

Additional Restorative Yoga sequences designed to gently nourish your body, reduce stress, and create an optimal environment to support fertility:

SEQUENCE 2

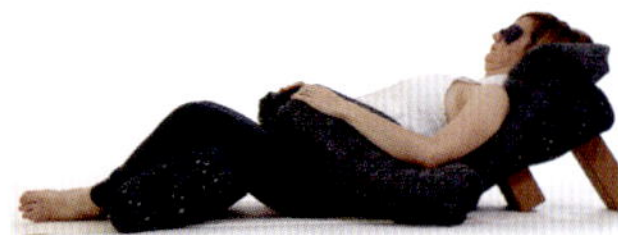

Supta Baddha Konasana (page 113)
10–15 minutes

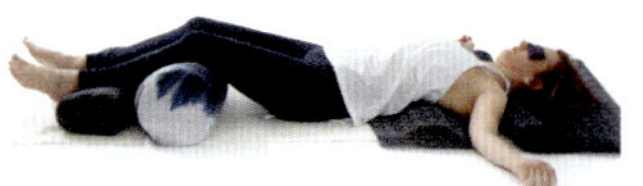

Salamba Matsyasana (page 31)
5–10 minutes

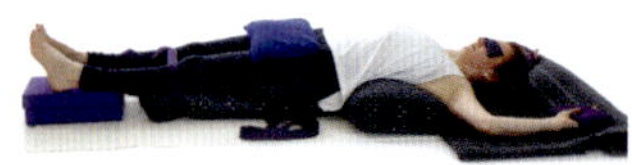

Salamba Setu Bandhasana with Straight Legs (page 94)
10–15 minutes

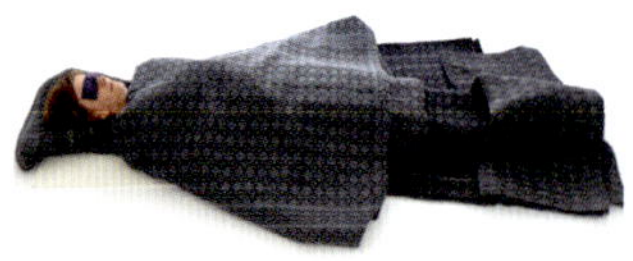

Swaddled Savasana (page 100)
20 minutes

SEQUENCE 3

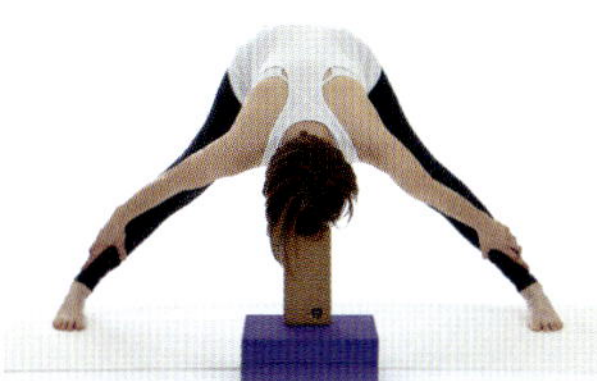

Salamba Prasarita Padottanasana with a Brick (page 176)
1–3 minutes

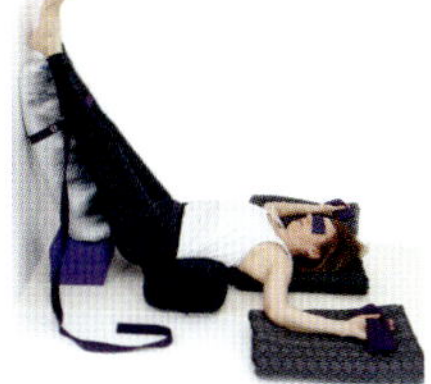

Viparita Karani (page 183)
15 minutes

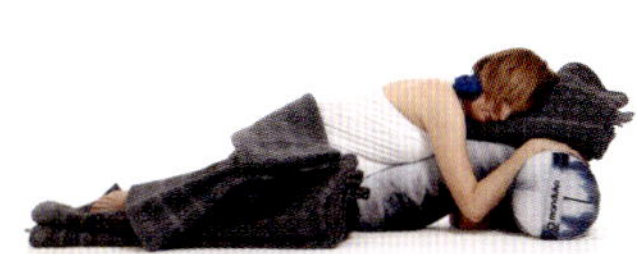

Salamba Bharadvajasana (page 53)
3–5 minutes each side

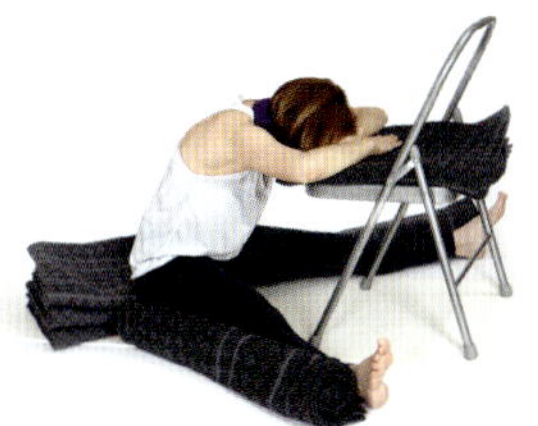

Salamba Upavistha Konasana (page 38)
3–5 minutes

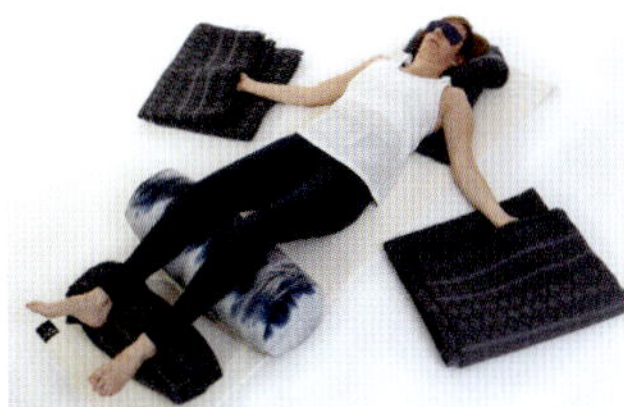

Salamba Savasana (page 41)
20–25 minutes

SEQUENCE 4

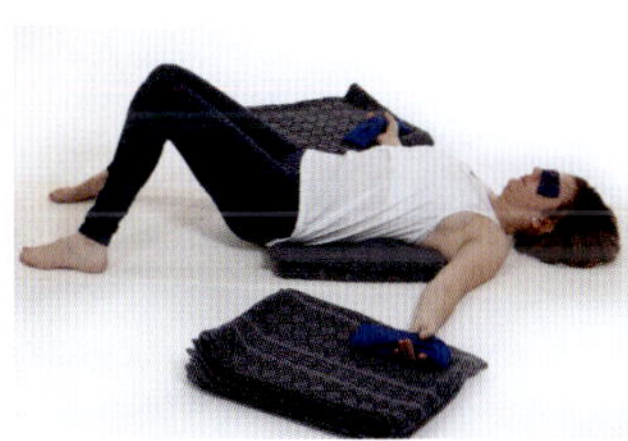

Salamba Urdhva Dhanurasana with a Blanket (page 91)
8–10 minutes

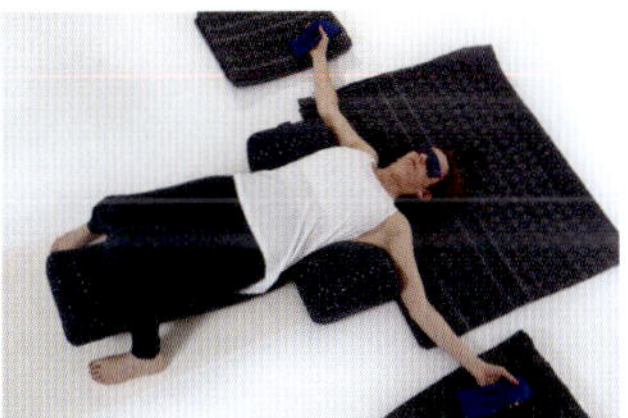

Salamba Setu Bandhasana with Bent Legs (page 97)
8–10 minutes

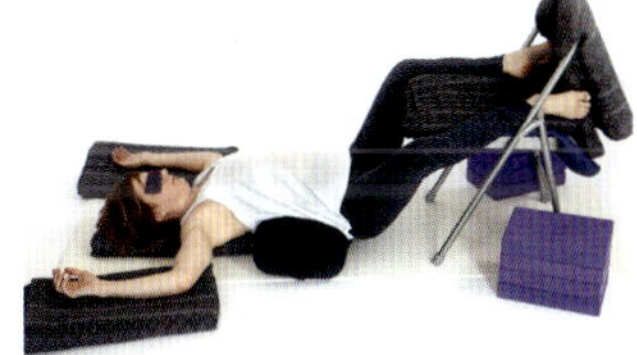

Viparita Baddha Konasana (page 138)
10–15 minutes

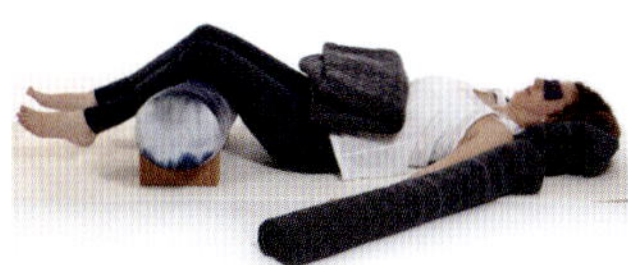

Savasana with Elevated Legs (page 187)
20–25 minutes

SEQUENCE 5 FOR ADVANCED STUDENTS

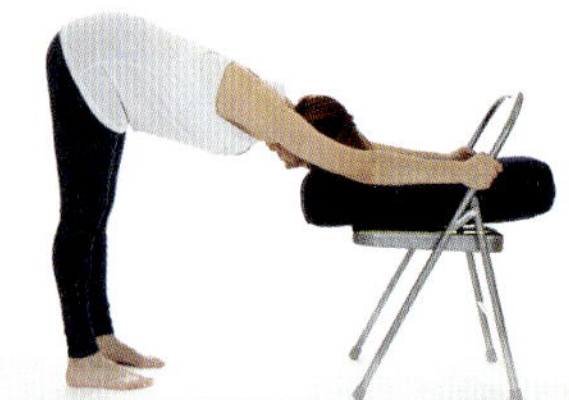

Salamba Adho Mukha Svanasana (page 180)
2–3 minutes

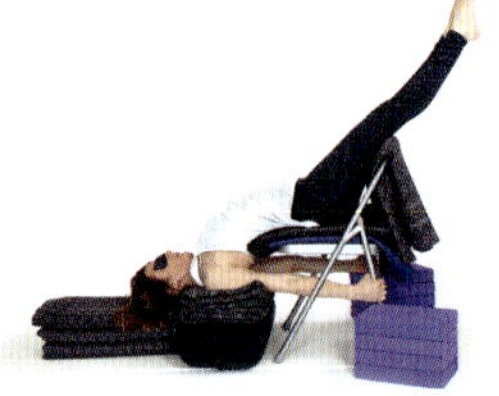

Salamba Sarvangasana (page 129)
5–12 minutes

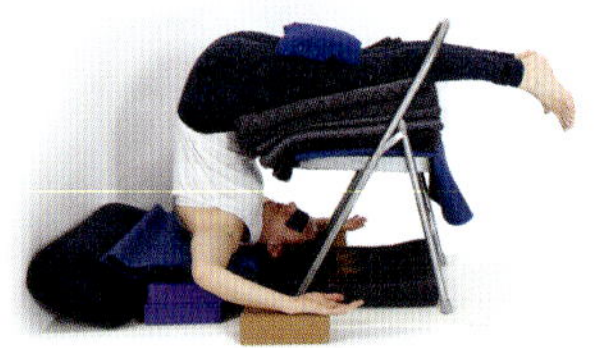

Ardha Halasana (page 141)
7–12 minutes

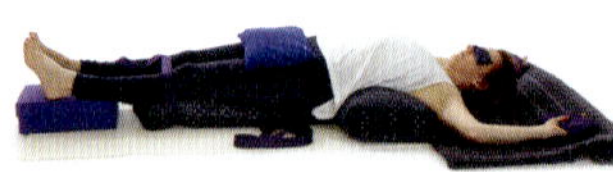

Salamba Setu Bandhasana with Straight Legs (page 94)
10–13 minutes

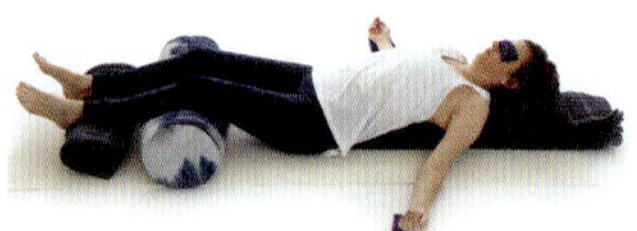

Savasana for Pranayama (page 60)
20 minutes

SEQUENCE 6 FOR IN VITRO FERTILIZATION AND AFTER EGG RETRIEVAL

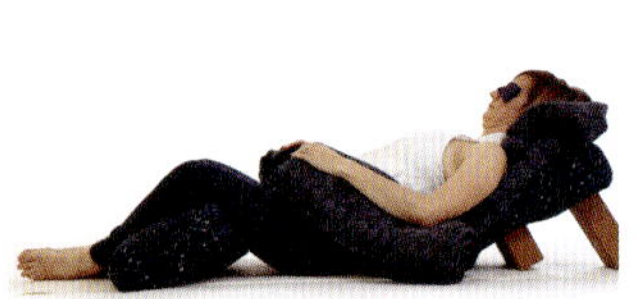

Supta Baddha Konasana (page 113)
15–25 minutes

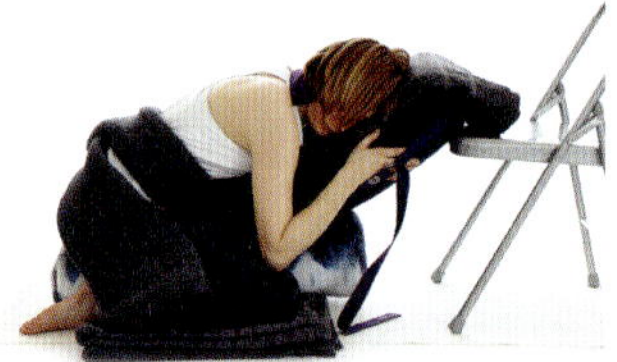

Salamba Balasana with Two Bolsters (page 116)
5–8 minutes each side

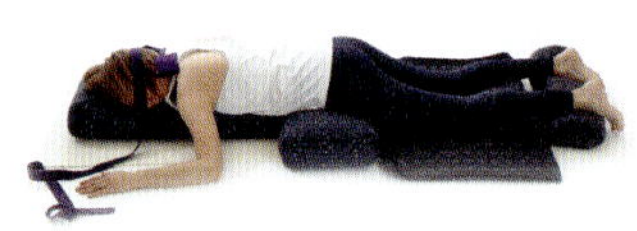

Adho Mukha Savasana with Two Bolsters (page 149)
20 minutes

Embracing Pregnancy and Childbirth

Pregnancy and childbirth can be emotionally and physically demanding, particularly for people who have faced challenges conceiving or experienced miscarriage. These experiences often bring heightened anxiety and vulnerability, but Restorative Yoga offers a gentle and effective way to reduce maternal stress and enhance mental well-being. This practice is especially beneficial for those with a history of infertility or loss, providing a nurturing space to foster connection with both the body and the growing baby.

During the early weeks of my first pregnancy, I was overwhelmed with anxiety, constantly worrying that every abdominal twinge might mark the end of my long-awaited journey. Restorative Yoga became my sanctuary. I vividly recall one practice during my third month when I was lying in Supta Baddha Konasana (fig. 4.1). In that tranquil moment, I felt an unmistakable sense of calm wash over me, as though my future child were reassuring me of his presence and encouraging me to trust. Even now, reflecting on this experience brings tears to my eyes. Throughout my pregnancy, whenever fear crept in, I would revisit that comforting memory and find solace.

In my second pregnancy, the challenges were different. Severe illness and fatigue marked the first trimester. Restorative poses like Salamba Supta Virasana (fig. 4.18) eased my nausea, while chest-opening poses improved my breathing and helped restore energy.

The Importance of Self-Care in Pregnancy

Every pregnancy is unique, unpredictable, and transformative. It often requires us to slow down and prioritize self-care for the health of both parents and baby. A pregnant person's emotional state directly affects the developing fetus; research shows that elevated stress or anxiety can influence the baby's heart rate. Restorative Yoga plays a vital role in calming the mind and balancing emotions, supporting hormonal regulation and helping to lower blood pressure.

Through gentle forward bends and poses inclined at a 45-degree angle, Restorative Yoga helps harmonize prana and apana energies, creating an internal environment of calm. Many of my students have shared that poses like Supta Baddha Konasana or Side-Lying Savasana (fig. 4.20) became invaluable during labor's early stages. These poses help expectant practitioners break the fear-tension-pain cycle. By fostering relaxation, they provide a sense of calm even during intense or demanding moments. Staying calm positively impacts the baby's health—panic can cause a drop in the baby's heart rate, potentially necessitating medical intervention.

From my personal experience, incorporating daily Restorative Yoga during my second pregnancy significantly reduced my post-cesarean pain and improved my recovery compared to my first delivery.

Postpartum Healing with Restorative Yoga

Restorative Yoga is just as valuable postpartum. After the birth of my children, I struggled with chronic sleep deprivation for over four years. Even when my children were sleeping peacefully, my nervous system remained on high alert, preventing me from achieving deep, restful sleep. A consistent practice of Restorative Yoga before bed gradually rebalanced my nervous system, and I eventually regained the ability to sleep deeply for up to eight hours.

The sequences I share in this chapter are designed to improve posture, relieve back pain, and address common pregnancy discomforts such as nausea, digestive upset, and water retention.

Avoiding Contraindications During Pregnancy

While Restorative Yoga is generally safe and beneficial, certain precautions are essential to ensure the safety and comfort of both the expectant practitioner and their baby.

INTENSE STRETCHING

Pregnancy naturally increases the hormone relaxin, which loosens connective tissues, ligaments, and tendons to accommodate the growing fetus and prepare for childbirth. While this added flexibility can feel empowering, it also increases the risk of overstretching. Overstretching can lead to permanent joint instability, particularly in the sacroiliac region, causing discomfort or pain. Similarly, overstretching the abdominal muscles can weaken their integrity, making postnatal recovery more challenging and increasing the risk of diastasis recti.

To avoid these complications, it's essential to remember that Restorative Yoga emphasizes gentle openings over intense stretching, with a focus on stability, balance, and ease. Always ensure that your body is fully supported in each pose, using props as needed to promote comfort and relaxation.

INVERTED POSES

During pregnancy, apana energy—the downward-flowing energy crucial for elimination—is naturally heightened to support pregnancy and prepare for labor. Inversions, which redirect this energy upward, are generally avoided in Restorative Yoga to maintain balance.

While modified inversions at a specific angle and for a limited duration can sometimes encourage a breech baby to turn, practicing these poses indiscriminately may increase the risk of complications. For example, inversions could inadvertently create a breech presentation or, in rare cases, cause the umbilical cord to wrap around the baby.[8] For most practitioners, it's best to avoid inversions during pregnancy unless specifically advised by a qualified health care provider.

LYING ON THE BACK AFTER THE FIRST TRIMESTER

After the fourteenth week of pregnancy, lying flat on the back poses risks due to potential compression of the inferior vena cava, the vein that returns blood from the lower body to the heart. This can lead to vena cava syndrome, characterized by low blood pressure, dizziness, and reduced blood flow to the placenta. To reduce this risk:

- Opt for poses that incline the upper body at a 45-degree angle.
- Side-lying poses are another safe and comfortable alternative, ensuring healthy blood circulation for both the expectant parent and the baby.

By understanding and respecting these guidelines, Restorative Yoga can be a powerful tool to nurture yourself during pregnancy, ease the challenges of labor, and support postpartum recovery.

Ardha Svanasana (Half Downward Dog Pose)

1–2 MINUTES

This pose effectively alleviates tension in the back muscles, releases tightness in the shoulders and hamstrings, and lengthens the spine. It also helps reduce fatigue by gently stretching and energizing the body. With regular practice, Ardha Svanasana can help relieve discomfort caused by round ligament cramps, a common issue during pregnancy, often triggered by sudden movements.

CONTRAINDICATIONS

- spondylolysis and spondylolisthesis

PROPS NEEDED

1 yoga mat, a wall

SETTING UP THE POSE

- Stand facing a bare wall, approximately 12 inches away.
- Ensure your feet are parallel to the edges of your mat and hip width apart.

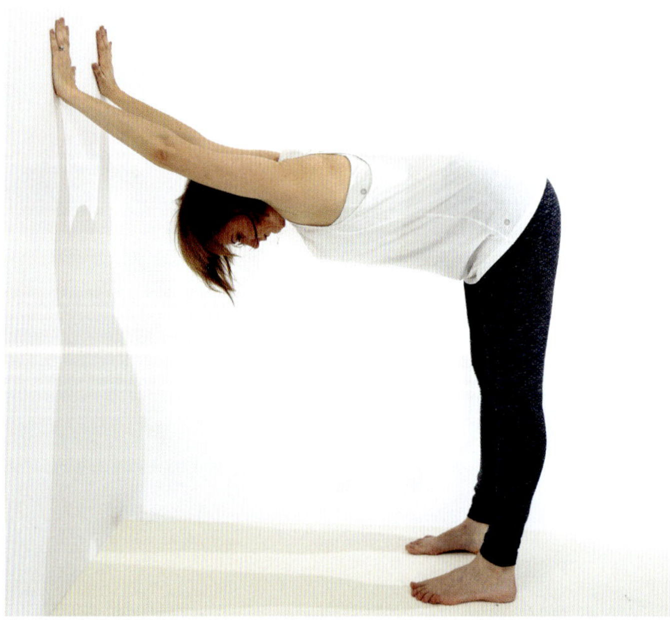

FIGURE 4.17 Audrey demonstrates a wall-supported Ardha Svanasana, creating a right angle at the hips to elongate the spine and gently open the shoulders and back body.

- Place your hands on the wall at shoulder height, shoulder-width apart, with fingers pointing slightly inward.
- As you exhale, slowly walk your feet backward while sliding your hands down the wall.
- Continue until your arms are fully extended, and your torso is parallel to the floor, forming an L-shape.
- If your back begins to round, adjust your hand placement higher on the wall to maintain a neutral spine (fig. 4.17).
- Lengthen through the spine, keeping your head aligned with your arms and gazing down.
- Keep your legs straight but avoid locking your knees by maintaining a slight micro-bend to prevent hyperextension.
- Actively press your hands into the wall, creating resistance.
- Simultaneously draw your femur heads (the tops of your thigh bones) back to lengthen your spine.
- Maintain this position for 1–2 minutes.
- Focus on deep, steady breathing, using each inhale to create space along the spine and each exhale to release tension.

ADJUSTMENTS FOR COMFORT

Hamstring or Lower-Back Discomfort

- Move closer to the wall to reduce the intensity of the stretch.
- Reposition your hands slightly higher, aligning them with your face, to reduce strain on your lower back and hamstrings.

Upper Back and Shoulders

- Maintain the natural curve of your upper back, avoiding excessive rounding or collapsing.
- If you feel discomfort in your shoulders, widen the distance between your hands to create more space.

Elbows and Knees

- Avoid hyperextending your elbows and knees. Keep a soft micro-bend in both joints to maintain proper alignment and prevent strain.

GUIDING STUDENTS THROUGH RELAXATION

During the practice, you can use the following guidance to help students relax deeply and connect with the pose:

- Close your eyes and breathe naturally. Sense the full weight of your body grounding through your feet as they gently sink into the earth. Imagine roots extending from the soles of your feet, anchoring you deeply into the ground.
- Feel your hands firmly pressing into the wall, as though your palms are merging with its surface. Visualize roots growing from your hands, embedding firmly into the wall, creating a sense of stability and connection.
- Maintain a natural and regular breath. With each inhale and exhale, imagine your breath traveling through an ever-growing trunk, your spine lengthening as your roots delve deeper.
- Let the warmth of your breath flow freely through your body, kindly releasing any tension along your spine, inviting relaxation to flow through your entire body.

TRANSITIONING OUT OF THE POSE

- On an inhale, step forward toward the wall, slowly lifting your torso upright to return to a standing position.

Salamba Supta Virasana (Supported Reclining Hero Pose)

8–15 MINUTES

Salamba Supta Virasana offers numerous benefits during pregnancy. By gently elevating the diaphragm, this pose creates additional space for the stomach and liver, thereby enhancing digestion and alleviating common issues such as morning sickness. Additionally, it expands the pelvic cavity, promoting optimal blood circulation within the uterus and accommodating the baby's movements. Regular practice can also help relieve constipation by stimulating the digestive system.

CONTRAINDICATIONS

- **knee injuries**: Practitioners with current or recent knee injuries should avoid this pose, as it places pressure on the knee joints.
- **ankle injuries**: Those with ankle injuries should exercise caution, as the pose involves flexion of the ankles.

PROPS NEEDED

1 yoga mat, 1 chair, 2 bolsters, 4–5 blankets, 1 yoga brick, 1 eye pillow

SETTING UP THE POSE

- Place a sturdy chair at one end of your yoga mat, facing you. If a chair is unavailable, position your mat in front of a sofa to utilize its seat as support.
- At the opposite end of the mat, lay two standard blankets widthwise to slightly lift your ankles. Tuck the thin edge under your ankle joints to reduce stiffness and provide adequate support for your feet and ankles.
- Position a round bolster lengthwise across the blankets. This bolster will serve as a seat, elevating your pelvis and reducing pressure on your knee joints.
- Place a second bolster at a forty-five-degree angle with one short end leaning on the first bolster and the opposite end against the edge of the chair or sofa.
- If the bolster is too soft, support it with yoga bricks to prevent it from sinking under your weight.
- Cover the second bolster with a single-fold rectangular blanket to provide extra comfort for your back.

- At the top of the bolster, add a standard-fold blanket folded into two layers: the higher layer should support your head, with the thickest edge placed under the C7 vertebra for optimal support, while the lower layer, with its thin edge, supports the top of your shoulder blades.
- Kneel astride the first bolster with your back facing the inclined bolster. Keep your legs hip width apart and your feet pointing straight back to maintain proper alignment and prevent strain on the inner knees. Let your shins rest on the blankets, with your feet extending just beyond their edges.
- Gently pull the calf muscles toward your heels to create additional space for bending the knees, reducing strain on these joints. Then lower yourself to sit down.
- Before reclining, ensure there is no gap between your seat and the second bolster for optimal support.
- Rest your torso on the inclined bolster and your head and shoulders on the supporting blanket.
- Adjust the blanket under your head, rolling its outer edges along the sides of your neck, head, and outer shoulders to provide complete support.
- Rest your hands gently on your belly, wrapping another standard blanket around your arms to support your elbows and forearms.
- Close your eyes and place an eye pillow over them to encourage deeper relaxation (fig. 4.18).
- Relax in this position for 8–15 minutes, focusing on slow, deep, even breathing to enhance the restorative benefits of the pose.

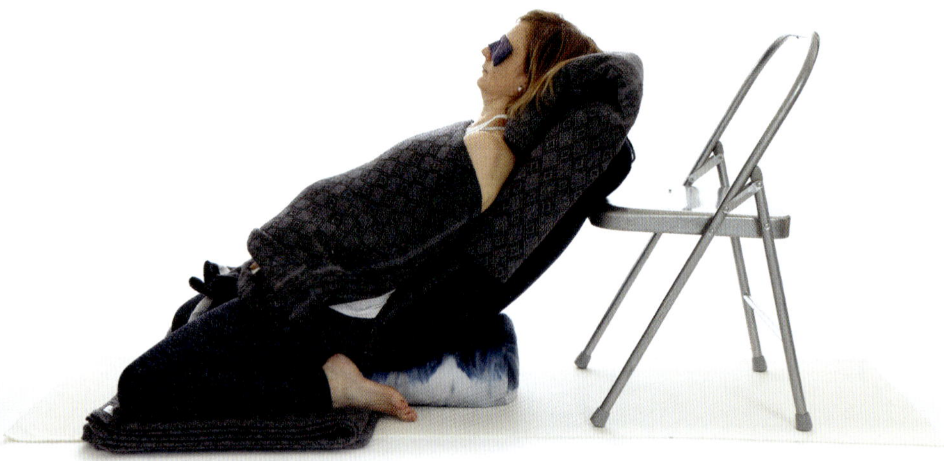

FIGURE 4.18 Audrey demonstrates Salamba Supta Virasana seated on a round bolster to reduce pressure on the knees and make the posture more accessible and comfortable.

GUIDING STUDENTS THROUGH RELAXATION

During the practice, you can use the following guidance to help students relax deeply and connect with the pose:

- Bring your awareness to your body. Allow the tops of your thighs to release and gently drop toward the ground.
- Breathe naturally, noticing how your legs grow heavier while your chest feels lighter with each breath.
- Visualize a refreshing stream of water flowing through your body, kindly washing away all tension. Imagine it cascading down the back of your head and neck, relaxing them completely as they sink deeper into the blanket. Feel the water flow down your face, softening any tightness in your eyes, ears, and mouth.
- As the stream moves over your shoulders and arms, let go of any stress or burden they carry.
- Feel it flow down your back, merging with the bolster supporting you, bringing a sense of unity and support.
- The stream flows through your chest and abdomen, bathing them in calmness and allowing them to relax fully.
- Finally, the water travels along your legs and feet, releasing any remaining tension. With nowhere to go and nothing to do, allow yourself to sink deeply into a state of complete rest, tranquility, and silence.

TRANSITIONING OUT OF THE POSE

- When it is time to come out of the pose, reconnect with the space around you by taking slow, deep breaths.
- Gently open your eyes and release your arms from the blanket.
- Place your nondominant hand under your skull, keeping the elbow close to your face.
- Position your dominant hand on the floor beside the bolster.
- Start by lifting your head, and then press your dominant hand into the floor to help you come to a seated position on your heels.
- Move onto all fours, and then slowly straighten your legs, walking your hands back toward your feet.
- With a slight bend in your knees, gradually stand up, moving with care and mindfulness.

Salamba Navasana (Supported Boat Pose)

15–20 MINUTES

Salamba Navasana gently opens the chest, enhances breathing, and creates more space for the stomach, reducing compression from the growing fetus. This pose is particularly beneficial for pregnant practitioners, as elevating the legs above the abdomen promotes lymphatic drainage and helps reduce swelling in the legs.

Incorporating Sama Vritti (Equal Breathing) during this pose can further enhance its benefits. This pranayama technique helps regulate the breath, minimizing spasms and tension during labor and facilitating the baby's delivery.

I encourage you to practice Sama Vritti to deepen your breathing while in this pose. Incorporate this breathing technique regularly in 45-degree-angle poses such as this one as well as Chaise Longue Pose (fig. 2.5), Salamba Navasana with Bent Legs (fig. 3.9), or Supta Baddha Konasana (fig. 4.1).

PRACTICING SAMA VRITTI PRANAYAMA

- Begin by observing your natural breath without making any changes.
- Gradually lengthen your inhales and exhales, ensuring the breath remains smooth and unforced.
- Alternate deep, extended breaths with normal ones to ease into a steady rhythm.
- Instead of focusing on counting, let your breath naturally extend based on your comfort level and inner sensations.

PROPS NEEDED

1 yoga mat, 1 chair, 3 bolsters, 1 yoga strap, 2 blocks, 2 bricks, 3 blankets, 3 eye pillows

SETTING UP THE POSE

- Start by placing an inverted chair at one end of your yoga mat. Lay a bolster lengthwise along the back of the chair to create a 45-degree angle (fig. 4.19).
- Cover the bolster and the floor with a blanket folded in half widthwise to provide extra comfort for your back.
- At the top of the bolster, add a standard-fold blanket folded into two layers. The higher layer should support your head with the thick edge placed under the C7 vertebra for optimal support, while the lower layer, with its thin edge, supports the top of your shoulder blades.

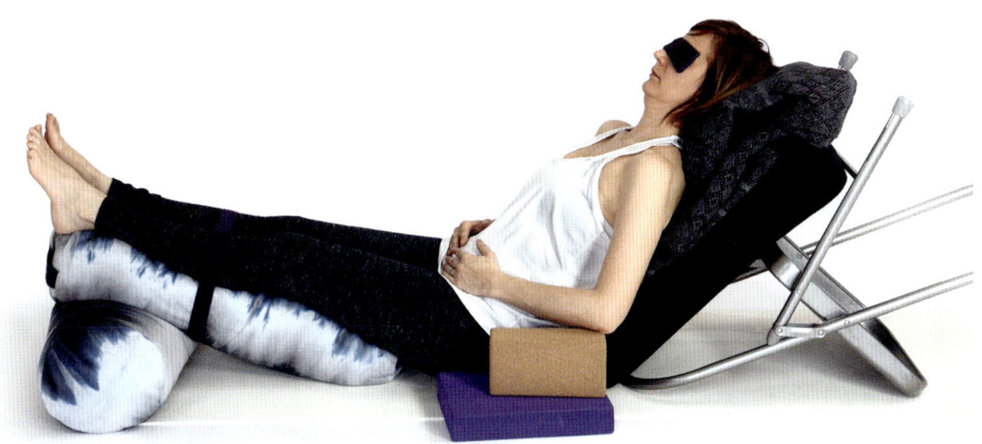

FIGURE 4.19 Audrey demonstrates Salamba Navasana with the torso supported at a 45-degree angle and the legs extended and elevated to promote rest and enhance circulation.

- At the other end of the mat arrange a second bolster widthwise. Position a third bolster lengthwise on top of the first.
- Sit in front of the first bolster and lie back onto it. Make sure there is no gap between your pelvis and the bolster to ensure optimal lumbar support and help open your sternal area.
- Rest your legs on the third bolster, internally rotate your legs, and buckle a yoga strap comfortably around your shins to encourage relaxation in your legs. Cover your legs with a blanket for warmth and comfort.
- Lie back and adjust the blanket under your head, rolling its outer edges along the sides of your neck, your head, and your outer shoulders to provide complete support.
- Rest your hands gently on your belly and support your elbows with a block and a brick on each side (fig. 4.19).
- Close your eyes and place an eye pillow over them.
- Relax in the pose for 15–20 minutes.

GUIDING STUDENTS THROUGH RELAXATION

During the practice, you can use the following guidance to help students relax deeply and connect with the pose:

- Begin by gently bringing your chin toward your chest, inviting a deeper connection with your inner world. Allow your body to release all tension.

Let your fingers curl softly. Release the muscles of your face and scalp, soften your belly, and allow your legs to surrender their effort in holding you up. Let your mind retreat inward, moving deep inside, like waves withdrawing from the shore.

- Shift your attention to your breath. Notice its natural rise and fall. The breath is an eternal mantra: always present, always available. As you inhale, feel the expansion of your back lungs, notice the lift of your side ribs, and then gently melt into the exhalation.
- With each inhale, open yourself to receiving. With each exhale, let go of all attachments.
- Begin to slowly lengthen both your inhale and your exhale. It's important not to force the breath, as this can tighten the diaphragm and create tension in your face and neck. Forcing the breath also stimulates your nervous system. To avoid this, just take a normal breath in and a normal breath out between each long inhale and exhale to rest.
- Take a long, slow inhale, reaching into the back body. Feel the back ribs expand, as we practiced earlier. Pause softly at the top of the inhale, and then transition smoothly into a steady, elongated exhale.
- Allow each breath to flow naturally, without jerking or forcing as you shift from inhale to exhale. Take a normal breath in and a normal breath out.
- Next take a long relaxed breath in. Feel the inhale begin in the back ribs, expanding the lungs as they open. Let the exhale begin in the lungs, imagining them gently contracting toward their center as the ribs follow, floating down softly.
- Keep your abdomen passive. Remember, the lungs are located in the rib cage, not the belly. Breathe into the back body, the side body, and the full rib cage, allowing it to flow and open. Inhalation is an act of reception; receive the breath fully. Exhalation is an act of release; feel the lungs gently squeezing inward and downward toward the center as the ribs follow.
- Take a natural breath in, followed by a natural breath out.
- Keep your abdomen completely passive throughout this process. Let your chin drop slightly to pacify the throat and maintain a sense of ease.
- Stay with this pattern for 5–7 minutes, alternating between deep expansive breaths and short pauses where you return to your natural breathing rhythm.
- After completing the deep-breathing cycle, allow your breath to return to its natural flow. Transition into relaxation, letting the calm you've cultivated ripple through your body, grounding you in stillness and peace.

TRANSITIONING OUT OF THE POSE

- As your relaxation comes to an end, gently bring your awareness back to the sensations of contact with the floor and the props.
- Observe your breathing: its quality, shape, and texture.
- Slowly remove the eye bag and allow your eyes to open softly, adjusting gradually to the light.
- Gently slip your legs out from the belt and bend one knee, then the other, placing your feet on the bolster.
- Inhale, and as you exhale, roll onto your side, resting on the bolster.
- When you feel ready, exhale and slowly return to a seated position, using your hands for support.

Side-Lying Savasana (Corpse Pose)

20–25 MINUTES

After the first trimester, lying on your back is not recommended because the inferior vena cava, located on the right side of the spine, may become compressed, restricting blood flow. Instead, resting on your left side is highly preferable.

In Ayurveda, the traditional holistic medicine of India, lying on your left side is thought to stimulate the digestive fire (called Agni in Sanskrit). This position directs more prana to the stomach and pancreas, which are located on the left side of the body. As a result, it can help alleviate common pregnancy discomforts such as nausea and heartburn.

In addition to its digestive benefits, Side-Lying Savasana supports deep relaxation and can be particularly helpful during the postpartum period. This position is ideal for breastfeeding, enabling the mother or birthing person to rest comfortably while nursing and fostering a sense of closeness with their baby. Personally, I found it invaluable with both of my children, as it allowed me to rest while they nursed and enjoy the comfort of close contact.

CONTRAINDICATIONS

If you experience pain in your left shoulder, consider lying on your right side instead, ensuring you are still supported and comfortable.

PROPS NEEDED

1 yoga mat, a wall or a sandbag, 2–3 bolsters, 4–6 blankets, 1 yoga brick, 1 eye pillow, 1 scarf

SETTING UP THE POSE

- Lay a yoga mat along a wall to provide a secure surface against your back. If desired, place one or two blankets on the middle of the mat for added cushioning and comfort. Position two or three double-fold blankets lengthwise at the top of the mat to support your head.
- Place a bolster lengthwise against the wall to support your back. If a wall isn't accessible, substitute with a sandbag behind the bolster or position yourself against the back of a sturdy couch for stability and a sense of security.
- Lie on your left side with your head resting on the prepared blankets. Adjust the height of the blankets to ensure your neck feels completely soft, and the top of your head tilts slightly upward. If needed, add another blanket under your head until the alignment feels comfortable.

- Place two single-fold rectangular blankets between your legs, extending from your knees to your feet. Alternatively, you can use a rectangular bolster. Your knees and feet should align at the same height as your hips to maintain a neutral spine and relieve tension in the lower back.
- Use your right hand to gently pull your left arm outward, creating space around your left shoulder and preventing the full weight of your body from pressing on it.
- Check that the bolster behind you remains firmly wedged between your back and the wall for added support.
- Place a yoga brick near the blankets supporting your head. Position a rectangular bolster at a slight incline, resting one end on the brick and the other on the floor near your thighs. This setup prevents any weight from resting on the arm beneath the bolster.
- Slide your left arm under the inclined bolster and rest your left wrist on a single-fold square blanket for comfort.
- Rest your right arm and hand on the inclined bolster. If your right elbow needs additional support, add a standard blanket lengthwise under your right arm, positioning it between your hip and armpit (fig. 4.20).
- Cover your body with a blanket to maintain warmth and encourage relaxation.

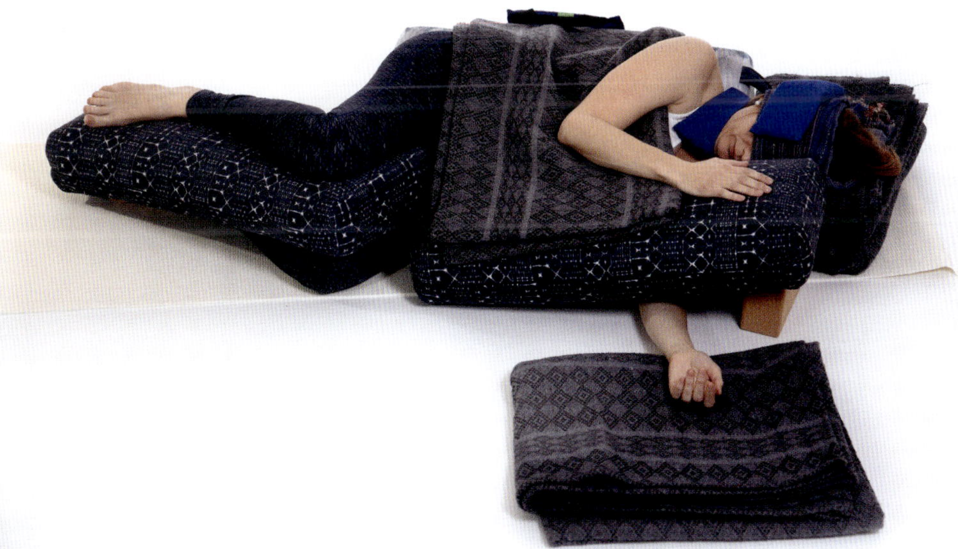

FIGURE 4.20 Audrey demonstrates Side-Lying Savasana with full-body support. The head, torso, knees, and ankles are cushioned for deep rest.

- Fold a scarf lengthwise and position it under your face, letting it gently drape over your eyes to enhance relaxation.
- Place an eye pillow at the back of your neck to support and relax your cervical spine.
- Add another eye pillow to the side of your forehead to help calm your mind and ease tension.
- Close your eyes and allow your body to relax completely. Rest in this position for 20–25 minutes, focusing on your breath and letting go of any tension.

GUIDING STUDENTS THROUGH RELAXATION

During the practice, you can use the following guidance to help students relax deeply and connect with the pose:

- Slightly lower your chin toward your chest and kindly scan your body with your mind. Slowly slide your awareness from your feet up your legs and into your pelvis and belly, chest, the top of your shoulders, arms, hands, neck, and head. With each exhale, release all tension.
- Breathe naturally through your nose, observing your body as it gradually relaxes and settles into the floor. Imagine your body as a hot-air balloon, releasing all its earthly tethers. With each exhale, feel physical and mental tensions dissolving, allowing you to rise effortlessly into the open sky.
- Sense your heart gently opening, as the warmth of your breath fills your chest, like the burners fueling the ascent of the balloon. Let this warmth spread, lifting you into a state of lightness and ease. If a swirl of emotions arises in your abdomen, welcome it with kindness. Offer it your full attention and compassion, surrounding it with gentle, loving energy, then kindly shift your awareness back to the sensations of your breath.

TRANSITIONING OUT OF THE POSE

- As your practice comes to an end, gradually become aware of the sensations of contact with the floor and the props.
- When you feel ready, gently remove the scarf covering your eyes.
- Mindfully disengage from the props, using your hands for support as you gently return to a seated position.
- Once in a seated position, with your eyes closed, take a moment to observe the effects of this practice on your body, mind, and emotions.

Restorative Yoga Sequences During Pregnancy

Additional sequences that can provide comfort and support during every stage of your pregnancy:

SEQUENCE 2

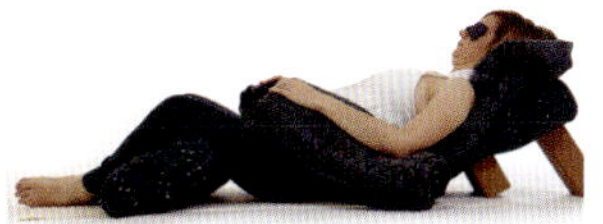

Supta Baddha Konasana (page 113)
20–25 minutes

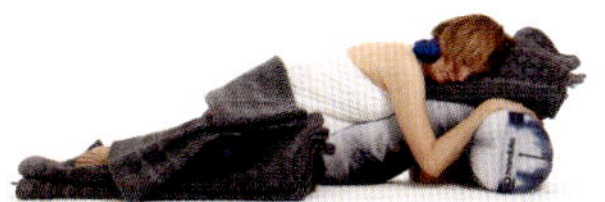

Salamba Bharadvajasana (page 53)
3–5 minutes each side

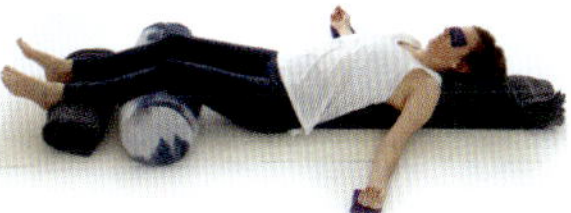

Savasana for Pranayama with Sama Vritti, until the end of second trimester (page 60)
20 minutes

SEQUENCE 3

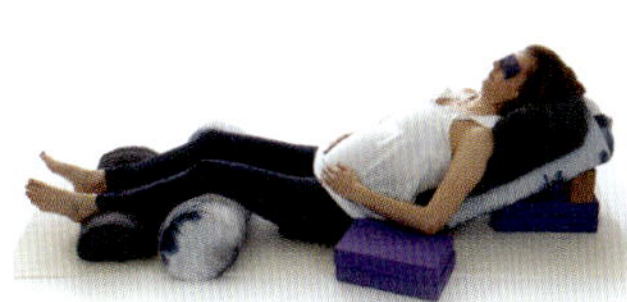

Chaise Longue Pose (page 28)
20–25 minutes

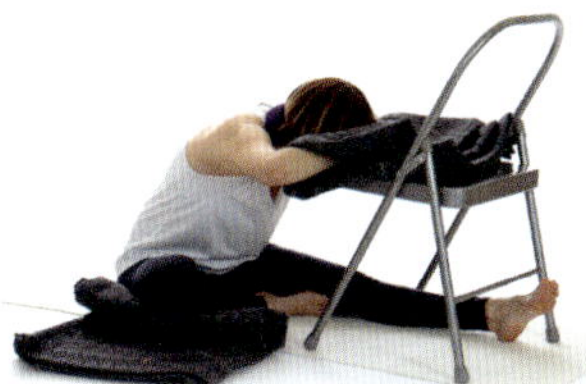

Salamba Janu Sirsasana (page 74)
3–5 minutes each side

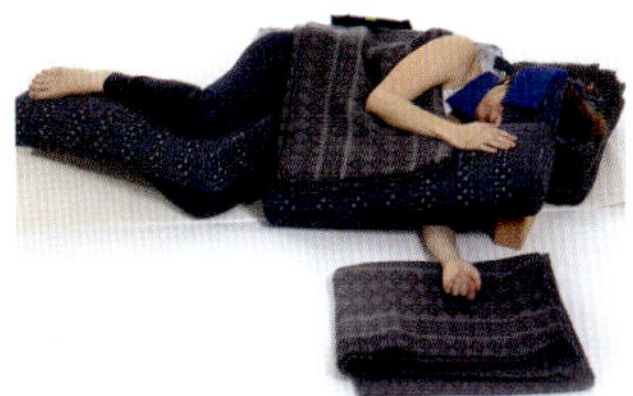

Side-Lying Savasana (page 168)
20–25 minutes

SEQUENCE 4

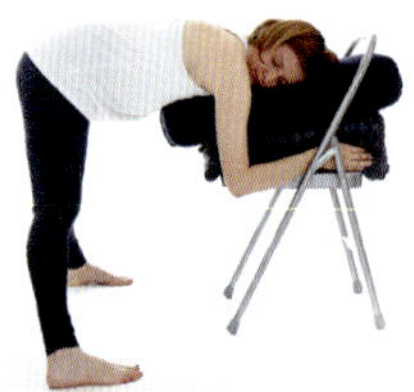

Salamba Prasarita Padottanasana with a Chair
(page 177)
2–5 minutes

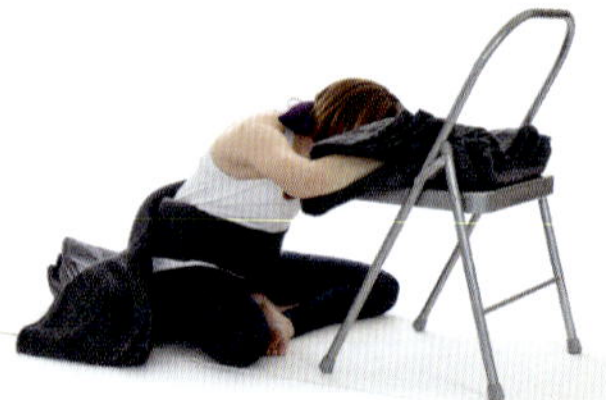

Adho Mukha Swastikasana
(page 50)
3–5 minutes

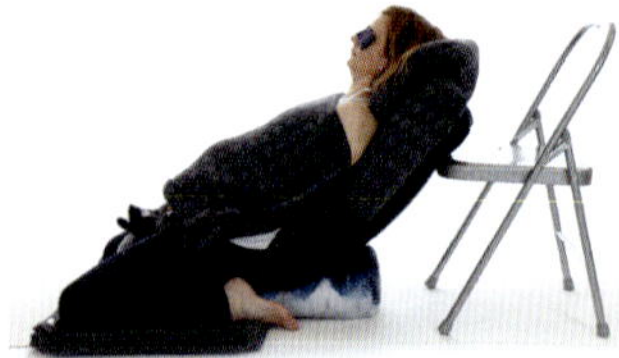

Salamba Supta Virasana
(page 161)
15–20 minutes

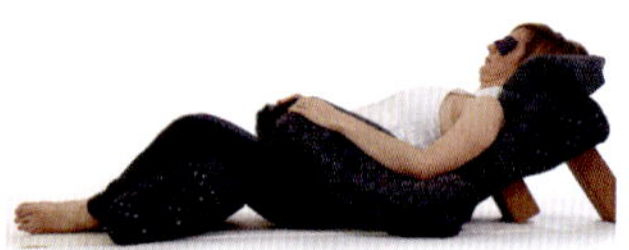

Supta Baddha Konasana
(page 113)
25–30 minutes

SEQUENCE 5

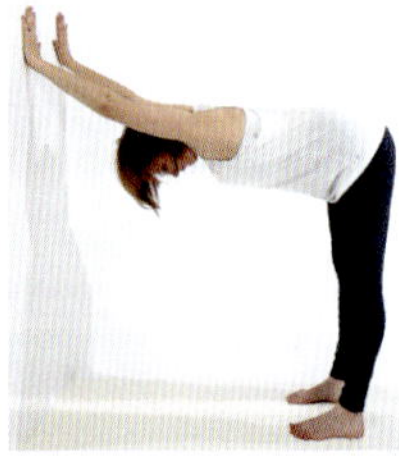

Ardha Svanasana
(page 158)
1–2 minutes

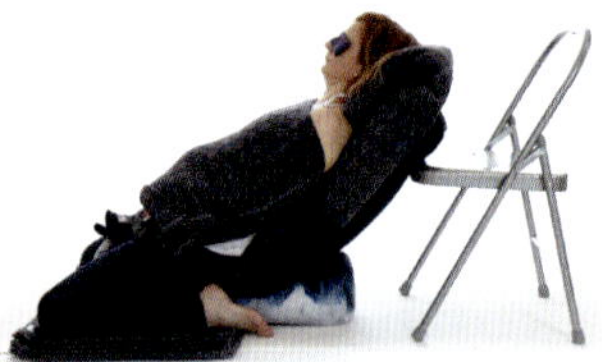

Salamba Supta Virasana
(page 161)
10–18 minutes

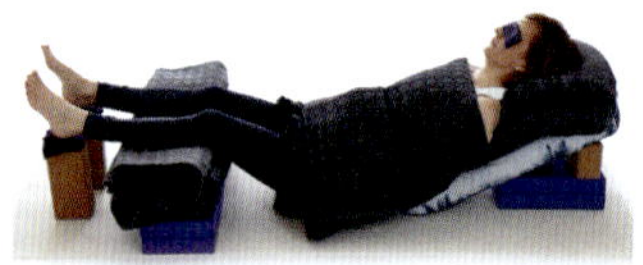

Salamba Navasana with Bent Legs (page 78)
15–20 minutes

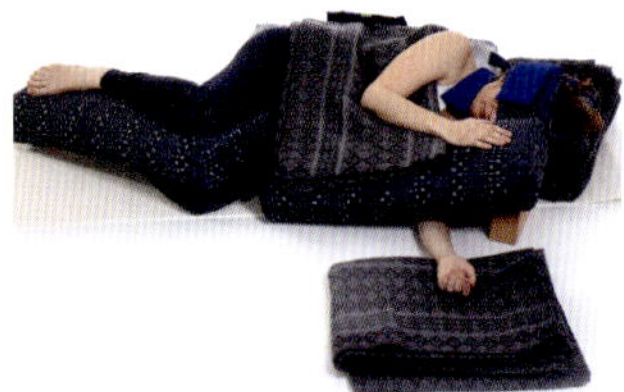

Side-Lying Savasana
(page 168)
20 minutes

Perimenopause and Menopause

Menopause, derived from the Greek words *mênos* ("month" or "menses") and *pausis* ("cessation"), marks the end of menstrual cycles. On average, menopause occurs around the age of fifty-two, though it can happen as early as forty or much later in some individuals.

Studies suggest that those with histories of trauma, whether physical, emotional, or sexual, may be more likely to experience early menopause.[9] This connection is believed to stem from how chronic stress reshapes the hypothalamic-pituitary-adrenal axis, accelerates hormonal depletion, and alters the body's long-term stress response. Trauma doesn't just reside in the mind; it lives in the body. It reshapes physiology, alters hormone production, and changes how we respond to stress over time. Chronic stress and unresolved inflammation gradually deplete the body's reserves, pushing the system into early transition.

The transition leading up to menopause, known as perimenopause, typically spans five to ten years, with significant variation in duration and intensity across individuals, ethnicities, and cultural backgrounds. Throughout this phase, the body moves through profound neurological and physiological shifts, driven by fluctuating levels of estrogen and progesterone. These changes can influence sleep, memory, emotional regulation, and overall well-being. At menopause, hormone levels drop by nearly 50 percent. By age eighty, DHEA, the hormone that helps buffer stress, may decline to just 10–25 percent of earlier levels.[10]

Hormonal fluctuations often give rise to a wide spectrum of symptoms: irregular periods, hot flashes, night sweats, disrupted sleep, and shifts in metabolism or weight. But the impact is not only physical. Emotional and cognitive experiences may also be affected, ranging from increased irritability and anxiety to brain fog and even depression. For some, these changes stir deeper questions of identity, particularly around purpose, visibility, and self-worth. These feelings often reflect not just internal shifts but also the social narratives we've absorbed over time. In many Western cultures, menopause is framed through a lens of decline. But alternative cultural perspectives remind us that this life stage can also be seen as a time of emergence, wisdom, and renewed authority. Recognizing and reshaping these narratives is part of the healing journey.

Importantly, no two experiences of perimenopause are the same. How we move through this transition is influenced not only by physiology but also by the emotional resources we've developed over a lifetime: our ability to regulate stress, our access to supportive relationships, and the degree of safety we've been able to cultivate within our own bodies. For those who've lived through chronic stress, trauma, or systemic adversity, this period may bring greater challenges. Conversely, those who have gently nurtured resilience and nervous system balance may find this transition more fluid.

Research into menopause highlights notable differences in symptom duration across populations. Vasomotor symptoms such as hot flashes and night sweats last an average of 7.4 years for white women, 10 years for Black women, 5.4 years for Chinese women, 4.8 years for Japanese women, and up to 12 years for those whose symptoms begin early in perimenopause. Black and Latin women, in particular, tend to enter this transition earlier, often in their thirties.[11] These variations remind us that menopause is not a uniform experience but a deeply individual journey influenced by biology, stress, culture, food, the gut microbiome, and access to care.

Meanwhile, other changes may continue to unfold well beyond the menopausal transition: shifts in bone density, genitourinary symptoms, joint pain, and increased inflammation are all part of the broader physiological reorganization that this life stage can bring. These longer-lasting effects remind us that menopause is not a single moment, but a process—one that continues to shape both the body and the psyche over time.

And yet, beyond the symptoms and statistics, this transition holds a deeper invitation. It can serve as a gateway into rest, clarity, self-awareness, and renewed personal power. At this stage of life, self-care is no longer optional; it is essential, and not as a luxury but as a profound act of honoring what your body has carried and what it is now asking you to receive. When met with compassion, knowledge, and support, menopause becomes not an ending but a rite of passage, a return to wholeness on new terms. Gynecologist and author Christiane Northrup describes it as a time of rebirth, a chance to redefine our purpose and embrace new beginnings.

For many, this stage of life also offers something essential, the opportunity to learn what we may not have learned before: how to take care of our nervous system, gently acknowledge the impact of past trauma, protect our yin energy, and nourish our vital reserves. These aren't abstract ideals; their effects are measurable, embodied, and deeply felt, influencing how we sleep, digest, think, and connect.

By supporting autonomic regulation and hormonal balance, we support:

- gentler menopause
- a stronger heart
- healthier bones
- life choices more aligned with our true energy and needs

The earlier we begin this preparation, the more we can support a smoother transition physically, emotionally, and energetically. Building this foundation over time allows us to meet menopause with greater resilience rather than urgency.

But preparing the body is only part of the journey. There is also a deeper invitation: to reimagine our way of living, to ask, What would it look like to live in rhythm with ourselves? This is the real challenge: learning to navigate the space between doing and being, between our drive to create, contribute, and achieve and our deep need to rest, receive, and slow down.

This is where Restorative Yoga offers not just support but sanctuary. It invites us to slow down deliberately, to listen inwardly, and to care for the body in ways that honor its natural intelligence—especially during menopause.

Restorative Yoga and Menopause

Emerging research highlights the role of Restorative Yoga in supporting menopausal well-being, particularly in reducing hot flashes. A pilot study demonstrated that Restorative Yoga is not only accessible to middle-age women, even those without prior experience, but is also highly beneficial. High rates of participant retention and satisfaction suggest that it is both well received and effective.[12] While more research is needed to understand the full scope of benefits, these early findings are promising—especially when paired with the lived experiences of countless practitioners.

Restorative Yoga supports the nervous and endocrine systems while awakening feminine energy (apana), fostering both physical and emotional balance. By creating space for deep relaxation and self-reflection, the practice helps shift perspective—from dwelling on what is passing to envisioning and actively shaping a life aligned with one's highest values.

To support this transition holistically, the upcoming yoga sequences incorporate gentle inversions, poses where the head is positioned below the heart, to assist hormonal regulation through the pituitary gland. These poses also help soothe hot flashes, enhance circulation, and invite a state of pratyahara (withdrawal of the senses), cultivating deeper self-awareness and inner calm.

Salamba Prasarita Padottanasana (Supported Wide-Leg Forward Fold)

1–6 MINUTES

Salamba Prasarita Padottanasana is a deeply restorative and supportive pose, particularly beneficial for practitioners navigating the transitions of menopause. By placing the feet wider apart than in Uttanasana, this standing forward bend offers a gentle and accessible stretch that soothes both the body and the mind.

This pose not only strengthens and lengthens the spine but also promotes flexibility and stability, providing relief from back tension. The mild compression created in this position soothes the pelvic and abdominal organs, enhancing hormonal health and encouraging improved circulation throughout the lower body.

The forward-bending motion naturally calms the nervous system, fostering a profound sense of inner peace while reducing stress. It also supports mental clarity, making it an ideal choice for moments of emotional or physical exhaustion.

As a gentle inversion, the head is positioned below the heart, increasing blood flow to the pituitary gland. This enhanced circulation can contribute to hormone regulation and help alleviate common perimenopausal symptoms, such as frequent or intense hot flashes, offering both physical relief and emotional balance.

CONTRAINDICATIONS

- herniated disc
- sinus infection or head cold
- pulled hamstring
- glaucoma
- retinal detachment

PROPS NEEDED

1 yoga mat, a selection of blocks and bricks

SETTING UP THE POSE

- Place a selection of blocks and bricks in front of you to adjust the height and support as needed.
- Stand with your feet parallel to the edges of your mat, about 3 feet apart. Remember, the wider your stance, the gentler the stretch on your hamstrings.
- Place your hands on your hips. As you exhale, drop your chin gently toward your chest and begin bending forward from your hip joints.

Maintain alignment of your head, lower ribs, and the front of your pelvis as you hinge forward.

- Rest your fingertips on the floor directly under your shoulders, keeping your spine parallel to the ground. Position the blocks or bricks under your head and adjust their height as needed to allow your neck to remain comfortably in flexion, avoiding any strain.
- On your next exhale, keeping your weight evenly distributed over your feet, fully lower your torso. Allow your lower back to round gently and rest the top of your forehead, at the hairline, on the blocks or bricks.
- Place your hands around your ankles. Ensure your hips remain aligned over your ankles. If you tend to overdo this pose in a more active practice, gently drop your tailbone toward your heels for a deeper release (fig. 4.21).
- Close your eyes and take slow, deep breaths. Allow your body to settle into the pose, feeling the gentle stretch and support. Soften your shoulders, jaw, and any areas of tension as you remain in the pose.

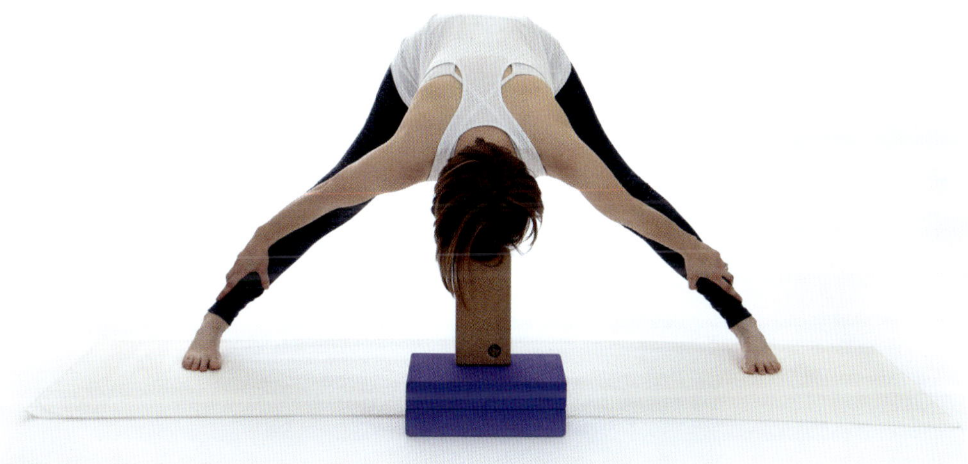

FIGURE 4.21 Audrey demonstrates Salamba Prasarita Padottanasana with the forehead supported on a cork brick placed on two foam blocks, a gentle grounding inversion ideal during perimenopause.

A MORE RESTORATIVE VARIATION OF THE POSE

Props Needed

1 mat, 1 chair, 2 blankets, 1 bolster, 1 eye pillow, 1 strap

Setting Up the Pose

- Place a sturdy chair in front of your mat and arrange a selection of double-fold blankets and a bolster lengthwise on its seat. These props will support your torso and head while you are in position.
- Stand in front of the chair with your feet parallel to the edges of your mat, approximately 3 feet apart. Place your hands on your hips. As you exhale, bend forward from your hip joints, maintaining alignment of your head, lower ribs, and the front of your pelvis.
- Rest your forearms on either side of the blankets on the chair. Gently allow your torso and head to settle onto the bolster. Turn your head to one side, your choice, ensuring your neck remains comfortable (fig. 4.22).
- If you experience any neck tension, place an additional eye pillow under the back of your cheek to reduce the strain caused by neck rotation.
- For deeper relaxation, you may also place an eye pillow at the back of your neck and use a strap to cover your eyes, as demonstrated in Adho Mukha Savasana (fig. 4.16).
- Close your eyes and relax in the pose for 2–3 minutes, focusing on your breath. Then turn your head to the opposite side and hold the position for another 2–3 minutes to maintain symmetry.

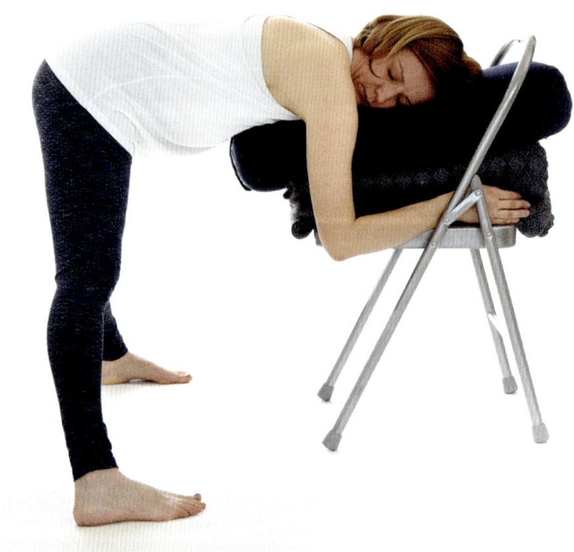

FIGURE 4.22 Audrey demonstrates a variation of Salamba Prasarita Padottanasana using a chair, a bolster, and blankets to promote grounding and gentle release of the nervous system.

GUIDING STUDENTS THROUGH RELAXATION

During the practice, you can use the following guidance to help students relax deeply and connect with the pose:

- Breathe naturally through your nose and gently bring your awareness to your body. Notice any areas of discomfort or tension. Let go of any judgment that may arise in response to this discomfort. Instead, direct your breath to that part of your body. With each inhale, breathe in compassion and nonjudgment. Observe what is happening right now. Perhaps, together, your compassion and your breath can begin to soften and ease that area.
- As you inhale, visualize bringing vitality and hope to this part of your body. With each exhale, imagine releasing judgment, doubt, and despair. In this way, you are actively cultivating self-compassion and nurturing yourself from within.

TRANSITIONING OUT OF THE POSE

- At the end of the pose, slowly open your eyes.
- When you feel ready, take a deep inhale and place your fingertips on the floor under your shoulders.
- As you exhale, bring your hands to the tops of your thighs to support yourself as you begin to rise. Move mindfully, but not too slowly, maintaining the natural curves of your spine throughout the transition.
- Once upright, pause briefly to stabilize your balance. Then gradually bring your feet together, allowing your body to return to a neutral and grounded standing pose.

Salamba Adho Mukha Svanasana (Supported Downward Dog Pose)

1–2 MINUTES

This restorative version of this standing pose offers significant physical and mental benefits, making it especially valuable during perimenopause. By gently inverting the body, it stimulates blood circulation, effectively combating fatigue and restoring energy levels. The supported alignment allows the back and shoulder muscles to release accumulated tension, fostering deep relaxation and a sense of ease.

The gentle stretch promotes diaphragmatic movement, enhancing breathing efficiency and expanding lung capacity, while the mild inversion of the head below the heart encourages increased blood flow to the pituitary gland, which may support hormone regulation. Additionally, the calming nature of this pose soothes the nervous system, helping to alleviate stress and ease tension-related headaches, providing both rejuvenation and tranquility.

CONTRAINDICATIONS

- sciatica
- sinus infection or head cold
- glaucoma
- retinal detachment
- spondylolysis and spondylolisthesis
- pulled hamstring (consider practicing Ardha Svanasana, fig. 4.17)

PROPS NEEDED

1 yoga mat, 1 chair, 1 bolster

SETTING UP THE POSE

- Place a sturdy chair at one end of a nonslip yoga mat. Position a bolster lengthwise on the seat to support your forehead during the pose.
- Stand facing the chair, approximately 12 inches away, with your feet parallel to the edges of your mat and hip width apart.
- Place your hands on the backrest of the chair, ensuring a firm grip.
- As you exhale, step back to a comfortable distance and bend forward from your hip joints, ensuring your spine remains elongated.
- Keep your feet parallel to the edges of your mat, distributing your weight evenly between them.

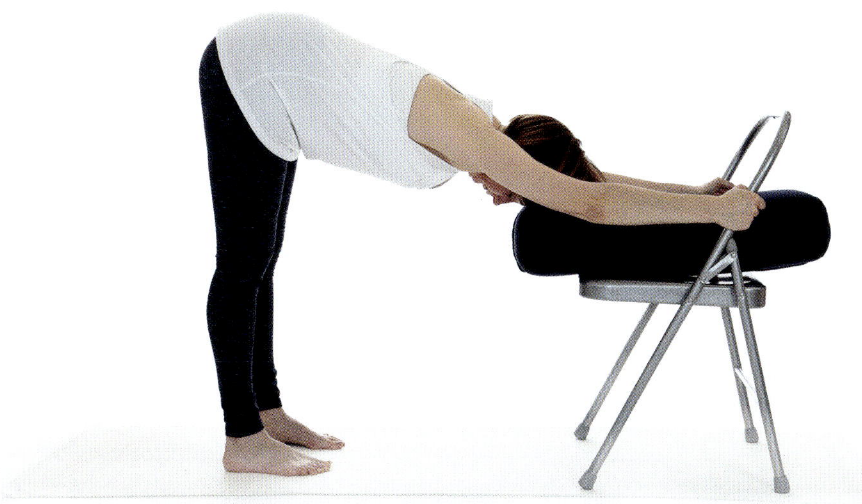

FIGURE 4.23 Audrey demonstrates Salamba Adho Mukha Svanasana with the head resting on a bolster placed on a chair to calm the nervous system. The hands press into the chair to create gentle spinal lengthening.

- Gently rest the top of your forehead, at the hairline, on the bolster, allowing your neck to relax in a flexed position.
- Carefully push the chair forward to create the classic Downward-Facing Dog alignment, ensuring its stability.
- At the same time, draw your femur heads (the tops of your thigh bones) back to lengthen your spine.
- Maintain a slight flexion in your neck, avoiding any arching (fig. 4.23).
- Close your eyes to enhance relaxation and internal focus.

GUIDING STUDENTS THROUGH RELAXATION

During the practice, you can use the following guidance to help students relax deeply and connect with the pose:

- Close your eyes and allow your breath to flow naturally. Feel the weight of your body grounding through your feet as they gradually sink into the earth. Imagine roots growing from the soles of your feet, anchoring you deeply into the ground.
- As you inhale, envision sap rising in your body, like a tree awakening from winter's rest.
- With each exhale, feel the sap flowing outward through your branches, preparing to bloom.

- With each inhale, sense the warm, revitalizing sap flowing through your trunk, infusing every fiber of your being with life and energy.
- With each exhale, imagine the first leaves gently unfurling, responding to the call of spring.
- As you breathe in, welcome the invigorating energy of spring into every part of your being.
- As you breathe out, visualize your branches expanding, with fresh tender leaves reaching toward the sky.
- With each inhale, feel your roots growing deeper, reaching toward the earth's center, connecting you to its powerful energy.
- As you exhale, sense the roots drawing up all the nourishment and strength you need to flourish.
- You are an oak tree, strong and generous, radiating a renewed sense of vitality and life.

TRANSITIONING OUT OF THE POSE

- At the end of the pose, slowly open your eyes.
- When you are ready, inhale deeply and place your fingertips on the seat of the chair for support.
- As you exhale, bring your hands to the top of your thighs to help you transition into a standing position.
- Move mindfully, maintaining the natural curves of your spine as you rise.

Viparita Karani (Legs Up the Wall)

15–20 MINUTES

Traditionally, Viparita Karani is more than a pose; it is a profound seal (*mudra* in Sanskrit), fully known as Viparita Karani Mudra. As described in ancient texts like the Hatha Yoga Pradipika, this mudra encompasses all inverted positions where the head is below the pelvis, such as Sarvangasana, Halasana, and Viparita Karani. This practice creates an energetic loop that circulates throughout the body, from the head to the feet, leaving you feeling deeply revitalized and restored.

Beyond its physical effects, this pose facilitates a connection with your inner essence, allowing you to transcend the physical body and access a profound sense of balance. It encourages a reflective state where your actions can align with your highest values, fostering harmony among the body, mind, and spirit.

CONTRAINDICATIONS

- pregnancy
- menstruation
- sinusitis or cold
- gastroesophageal reflux
- spondylolysis and spondylolisthesis
- glaucoma
- retinal detachment
- for tight hamstrings, practice Ardha Viparita Karani (fig. 3.3)

PROPS NEEDED

1 yoga mat, a wall, 2 bolsters, 1 strap, 4 blankets, several blocks, 3 eye pillows

SETTING UP THE POSE

- Place a yoga mat perpendicular to the wall. Position a bolster horizontally about 12 inches from the wall. Insert several blocks between the wall and the bolster to create a firm foundation, and place a second bolster vertically on top of these blocks to support your legs. This setup helps prevent hyperextension of the knee joints. Secure the second bolster loosely with a yoga strap to keep your legs stable throughout the pose.

- Place a double-fold blanket lengthwise in front of the horizontal bolster to support your shoulders and head. Keep two extra blankets nearby to cushion your forearms once you are in position.
- Sit on your heels at one end of the horizontal bolster, facing the center of the room. Align the outer edge of your hip with the middle of the bolster. If the bolster is on your right, lean forward, bringing your chest toward your thighs, and extend your right arm across your chest. Inhale deeply, and as you exhale, roll over onto your back and swing your legs up onto the vertical bolster. Place your legs, one at a time, between the bolster and the strap for added stability.
- Rest your pelvis and lower ribs on the horizontal bolster, while your shoulders and head are supported by the blanket.
- Ensure your lower ribs are well supported by the bolster, creating a gentle backbend. This slight backbend stimulates the abdominal organs, particularly the lower ones.
- Position your pubic bone level with or slightly lower than your navel. This gentle opening in the front of the pelvis encourages improved blood flow to the reproductive organs, providing them with oxygen and nutrients to support optimal function.

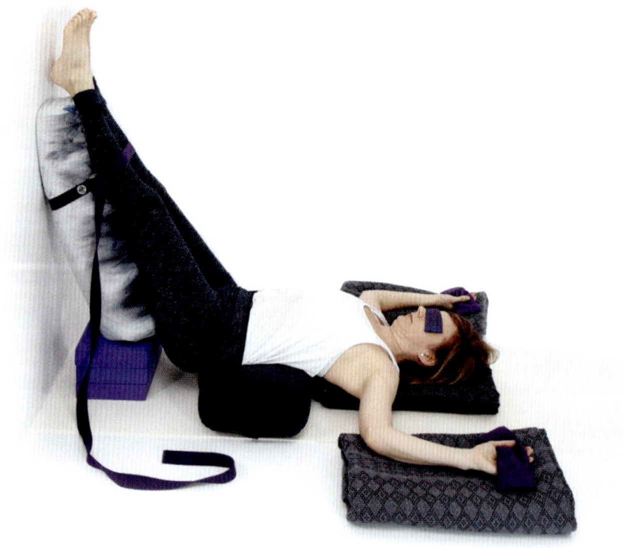

FIGURE 4.24 Audrey demonstrates Viparita Karani with the pelvis on a bolster and a second bolster placed against the legs to prevent hyperextension of the knees.

- Ensure that your thighs are inclined at an angle greater than 90 degrees relative to the floor to release tension in the thighs, psoas muscles, and abdomen. The bolster should support the fullest part of your calves and thighs, ensuring full relaxation of the legs. Rotate your lower legs inward slightly and secure your shins firmly with the strap for stability.
- Choose the arm position that feels most comfortable for you:
  - Extend your arms overhead (fig. 4.24) to release tension in the trapezius and deltoid muscles.
  - Position your arms alongside your body, as in Ardha Viparita Karani for a more grounded variation (fig. 3.3).
- Place an eye pillow in the palm of each hand for added comfort. Cover yourself with a blanket, close your eyes, and gently place another small eye pillow over them to block out light and encourage deeper relaxation.
- Remain in this position for 15–20 minutes. If you experience any tingling or numbness in your feet, it is a signal to gently come out of the pose.

GUIDING STUDENTS THROUGH RELAXATION

During the practice, you can use the following guidance to help students relax deeply and connect with the pose:

- Bring your awareness to your body. Notice all the places where your body connects with the props supporting you. Take several deep breaths, allowing yourself to progressively release all tension. Trust the props and the wall to hold you completely.
- Release any tension in your legs and pelvis. Let go of any gripping or holding.
- Invite ease into your chest, shoulders, head, and neck. Feel these areas soften as you settle further into stillness.
- Shift your focus to the natural rhythm of your breath without trying to control it. Direct your attention to the subtle rise and fall of your chest. As you inhale, feel your lower ribs expand; as you exhale, notice the gentle echo of movement in the back of your body.
- With each breath in, feel the movement of each rib outward and upward. As you breathe out, notice the gradual relaxation of your chest muscles and the gentle contraction of your rib cage—a soft, rhythmic symphony.
- Now, visualize a butterfly resting where your chest resides. With each inhale, imagine your lungs expanding into the vibrant wings of a multicolored butterfly taking flight.

- Your relaxed belly follows this gentle rhythm. Allow the muscles of your face to release tension—the outer jaw and the root of your tongue soften. Your arms and legs are completely at rest. Every cell in your body inhales and exhales in harmony, radiating calm and balance.
- Feel your body growing lighter, as if levitating. The butterfly's wings begin to transform, becoming light and translucent, like an angel's wings.
- As you rest here, feel deeply connected to your inner essence—fully at peace in the present moment.

TRANSITIONING OUT OF THE POSE

- As your relaxation comes to an end, reconnect with the space around you by taking slow, deep breaths.
- Remove your eye pillow and carefully release your legs from the strap.
- Slowly slide off the bolster until your entire back rests flat on the floor.
- Bend your knees and remain in this position for a few moments.
- When you feel ready, roll onto your side and return to a seated position.

Savasana (Corpse Pose) with Elevated Legs

25–30 MINUTES

This variation of Savasana elevates the legs above the heart, offering a gentle inversion that promotes multiple benefits:

- **enhanced blood circulation**: Encourages venous return from the legs to the heart, reducing swelling and fatigue.
- **lymphatic drainage**: Supports the detoxification process by facilitating lymph flow through the legs and abdominal organs.
- **relaxation of the psoas and lower back**: The positioning and angle of the legs help release tension in the psoas muscles and ease strain on the lower back, fostering a deep state of relaxation.

CONTRAINDICATIONS

- **menstruation**: Practice Savasana with Elevated and Weighted Ankles (fig. 4.5).
- **pregnancy (after the first trimester)**: Avoid lying flat on the back. Instead, opt for Side-Lying Savasana on the left side to ensure optimal blood flow to the baby and to prevent discomfort (fig. 4.20).

PROPS NEEDED

1 yoga mat, 1 bolster, 2 yoga bricks, 5 blankets, 1 eye pillow

SETTING UP THE POSE

- Sit on your mat with your knees bent and your feet flat on the ground.
- Fold a standard blanket into two layers and place it horizontally at the top of your mat. The higher layer should support your head, with the thick edge placed under the C7 vertebra for optimal support, while the lower layer, with its thin edge, supports the top of your shoulder blades. Roll the blanket's edges gently to cradle the sides of your neck, head, and outer shoulders for full support.
- Place a bolster under your knees, supported by two bricks to elevate the legs. Cover your legs with a blanket.
- Adjust the bolster and bricks so that your thighs rest at a 45-degree angle to the floor, ensuring the backs of your knees are fully supported and your feet are slightly lower than your knees for maximum relaxation.

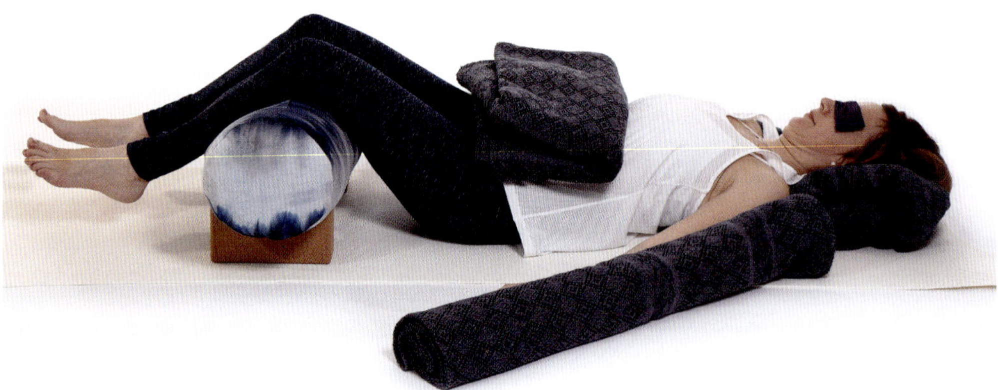

FIGURE 4.25 Audrey demonstrates a variation of Savasana with the legs elevated and at a 45-degree angle, knees higher than the feet, to enhance venous return and support the lower back.

- Lie back comfortably, allowing your arms to rest at a minimum 45-degree angle from your torso. Let your elbows relax on the ground, with your palms gently facing toward your body, resting on your little fingers. For a cocooned and supported sensation, you can place a rolled blanket lengthwise along each arm.
- On an exhale, place a single-fold square blanket over your navel area to help relax your abdomen and lower back (fig. 4.25).
- Gently release the base of your head, inviting a sense of calm and mental stillness.
- Fully cover yourself with a blanket, close your eyes, and place an eye pillow over them. Relax in this position for 25–30 minutes.

GUIDING STUDENTS THROUGH RELAXATION

During the practice, you can use the following guidance to help students relax deeply and connect with the pose:

- Gently bring your awareness to your body. Slowly scan your body with your mind, sensing all the places where it connects with the props and the ground, from your feet to your head.
- Begin by noticing where your legs meet the supports. With each exhale, allow them to release fully, sinking farther into the bolster.
- Shift your attention to your sacrum and lower back. With every exhale, let them settle deeper into the earth, and feel your belly softening as it gently rests into your back.

- Move your focus to your back. Let it melt into the ground, feeling the earth's support spreading around you.
- Bring your awareness to your head, neck, and shoulders. Allow these areas to be completely held by the ground, releasing all tension.
- Let your arms and hands relax completely, resting in the earth's support.
- Feel the earth holding you, wrapping you in softness. Notice your breath deepen as you trust and rely on its unconditional support.

TRANSITIONING OUT OF THE POSE

- As your practice comes to an end, begin to reconnect with the space around you by taking slow, deep breaths.
- When you feel ready, exhale while keeping your lower back and pelvis stable, and slowly draw one knee toward your chest, followed by the other.
- Roll onto the side of your choice, allowing your eye pillow to fall softly to the ground. Rest here for a few breaths.
- At your own pace, press the hand closest to your chest into the floor, using the other for support, and gently return to a seated position.
- With your eyes still closed, take a few moments to observe the effects of this sequence on your body, mind, and emotions. Observe any changes with curiosity and without judgment.

Restorative Yoga Sequences for Menopause

Explore these additional Restorative Yoga sequences tailored to nurture your body and mind during the significant transitions of menopause. These carefully crafted practices help alleviate common symptoms, promote hormonal balance, and offer a soothing space for relaxation and self-care as you navigate this transformative stage of life.

SEQUENCE 2

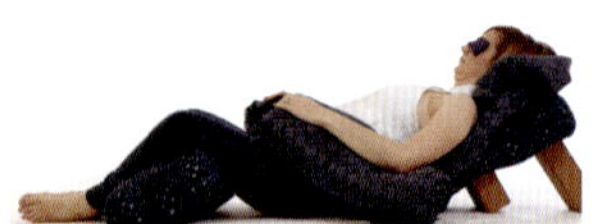

Supta Baddha Konasana (page 113)
15–20 minutes

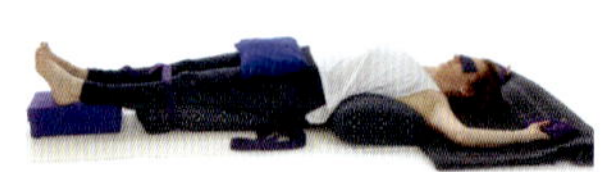

Salamba Setu Bandhasana with Straight Legs (page 94)
10–15 minutes

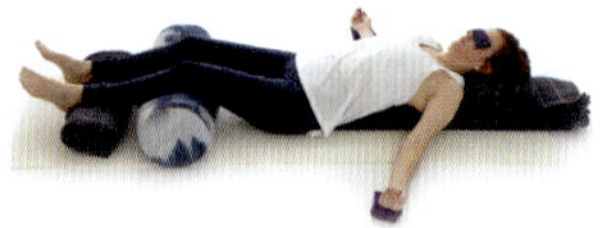

Savasana for Pranayama (page 60)
20–25 minutes

SEQUENCE 3

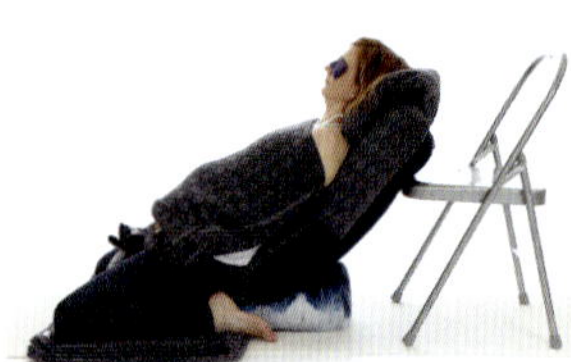

Salamba Supta Virasana (page 161)
10–15 minutes

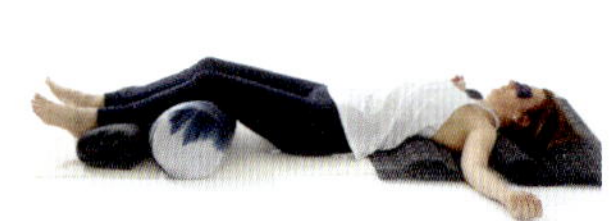

Salamba Matsyasana (page 31)
10 minutes

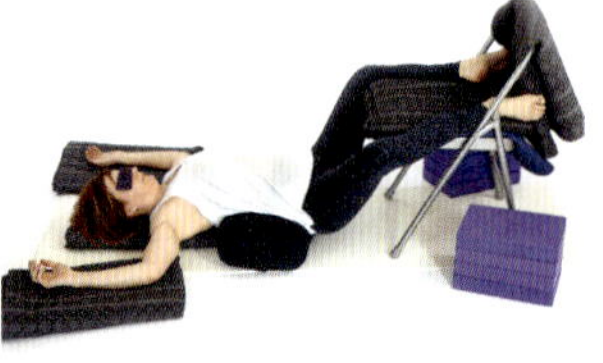

Viparita Baddha Konasana (page 138)
10–15 minutes

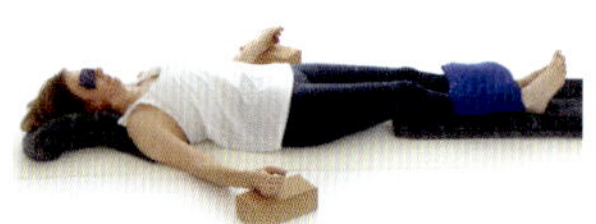

Savasana with Elevated and Weighted Ankles (page 122)
15–20 minutes

SEQUENCE 4

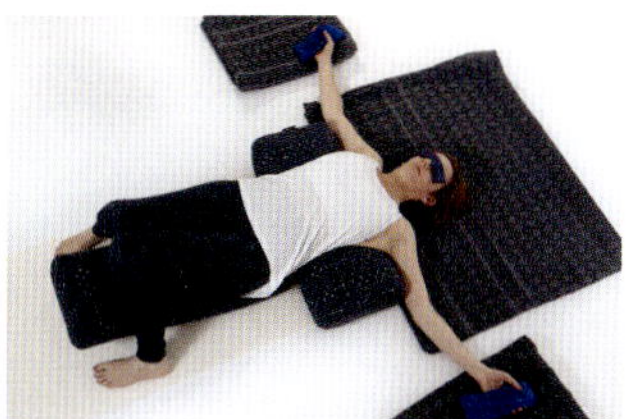

Salamba Setu Bandhasana with Bent Legs (page 97)
8–10 minutes

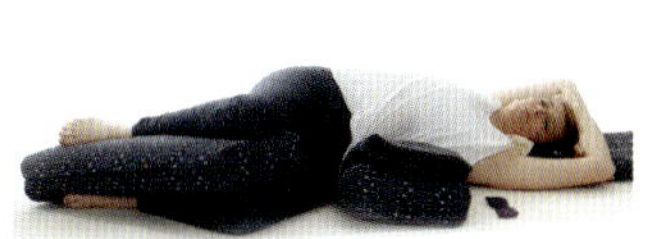

Salamba Jathara Parivartanasana (page 35)
2–3 minutes each side

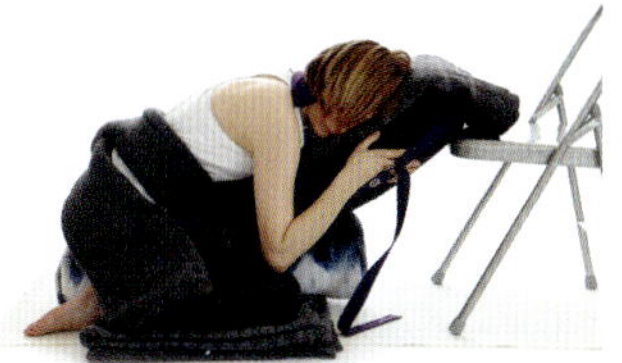

Salamba Balasana with Two Bolsters (page 116)
2–3 minutes each side

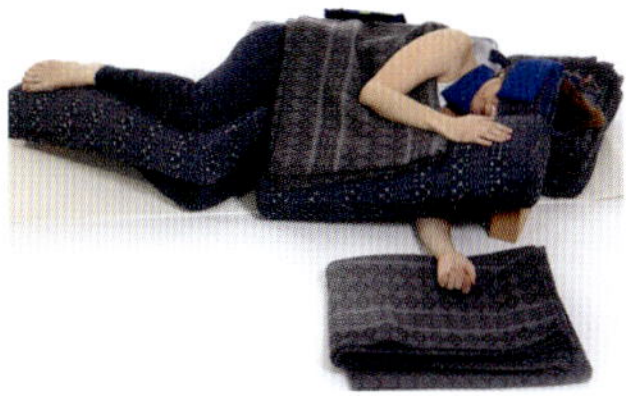

Side-Lying Savasana (page 168)
15–20 minutes

SEQUENCE 5 FOR ADVANCED STUDENTS

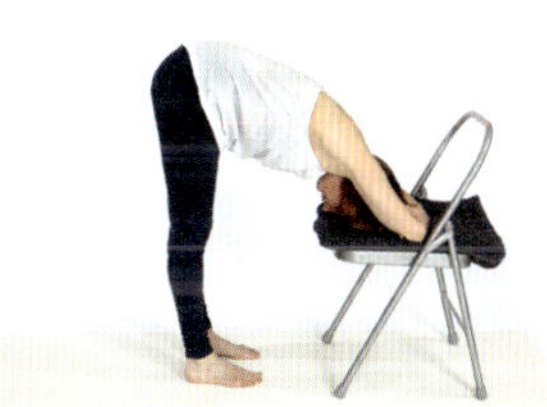

Salamba Uttanasana (page 71)
2–3 minutes

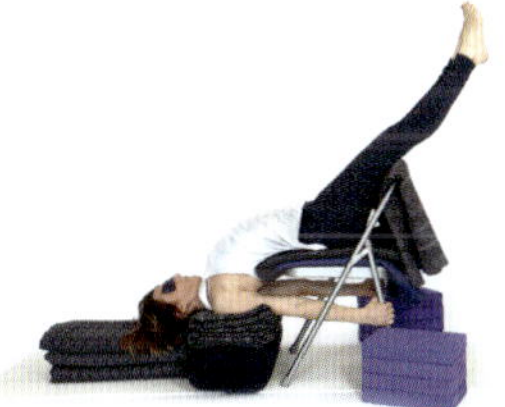

Salamba Sarvangasana (page 129)
5–10 minutes

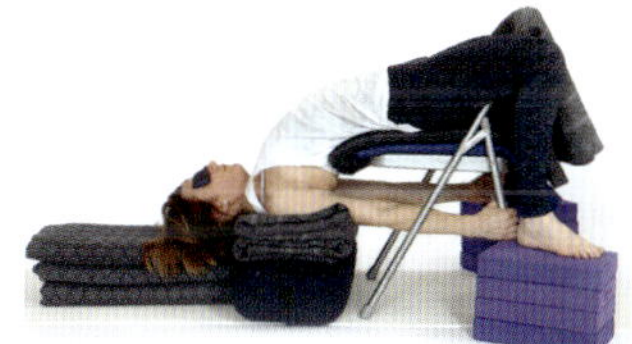

Salamba Urdhva Dhanurasana with a Chair (page 135)
5 minutes

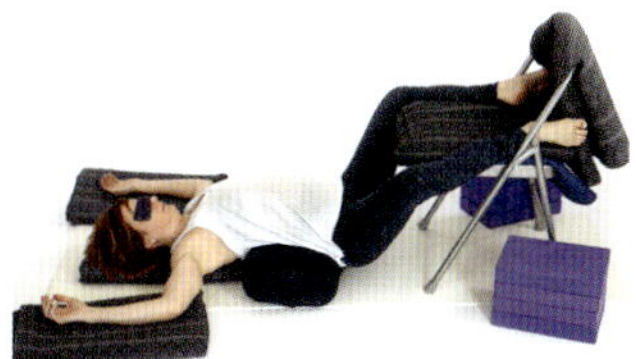

Viparita Baddha Konasana (page 138)
15–20 minutes

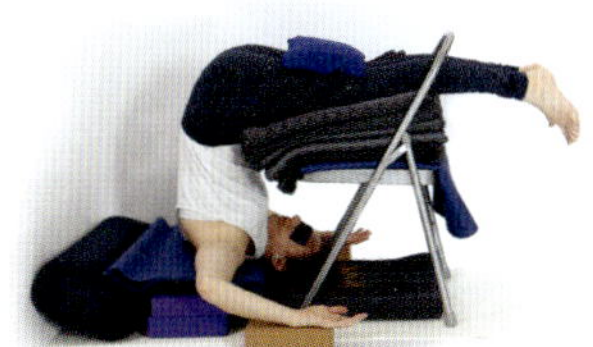

Ardha Halasana (page 141)
5–10 minutes

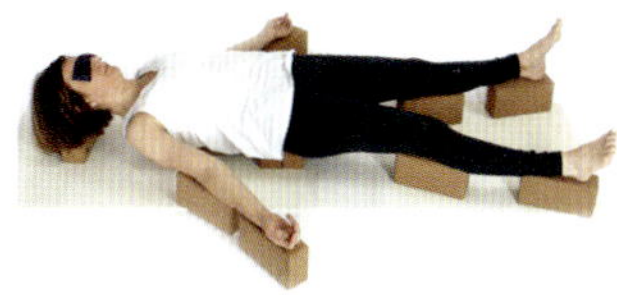

Bhishmasana (page 83)
12 minutes

Conclusion

Our lives are often dominated by yang energy, the solar, outward, and active force that drives productivity, ambition, and growth. While this energy is vital, it can overshadow its equally important counterpart, yin energy. Yin represents the quieter, introspective, and receptive qualities, the lunar and feminine principle of the universe. To achieve true emotional balance and unlock our full potential, we must honor and cultivate both energies.

Restorative Yoga offers a profound invitation to embrace yin energy and the art of slowing down. This practice is not about stepping away from action but enriching it with intention, meaning, and presence. By allowing ourselves to pause and rest, we create space for creativity to thrive, emotional clarity to unfold, and more compassionate connections to take root and flourish.

Just twenty minutes of intentional rest each day can transform not only how we feel but how we show up in the world. It reminds us that rest is not a luxury; it's a necessity. Through this mindful practice, we can contribute to a calmer, more empathetic, and harmonious world, one breath at a time.

Resources

Books

YOGA

Bo Forbes, *Yoga for Emotional Balance: Simple Practices to Help Relieve Anxiety and Depression* (Shambhala, 2011)
Gita S. Iyengar, *Yoga: A Gem for Women* (1983)
Jillian Pransky, *Deep Listening: A Healing Practice to Calm Your Body, Clear Your Mind, and Open Your Heart* (Rodale, 2017)
Judith Hanson Lasater, *Relax and Renew: Restful Yoga for Stressful Times* (Rodmell, 1995; repr. Shambhala, 2016)
Judith Hanson Lasater, *Restore and Rebalance: Yoga for Deep Relaxation* (Shambhala, 2017)
Judith Hanson Lasater, *Yoga Myths: What You Need to Learn and Unlearn for a Safe and Healthy Yoga Practice* (Shambhala, 2020)
Mel Robin, *A Physiological Handbook for Teachers of Yogasana* (Fenestra, 2002)
Silva Mehta, Mira Mehta, and Shyam Mehta, *Yoga the Iyengar Way: The New Definitive Illustrated Guide* (Knopf, 1990)

YOGA PHILOSOPHY

Hatha Yoga Pradipika
Judith Hanson Lasater and Ike Lasater, *What We Say Matters: Practicing Nonviolent Communication* (Shambhala, 2009)

ANATOMY

Judith Hanson Lasater, *Yogabody: Anatomy, Kinesiology and Asana* (Shambhala, 2009)

HEALTH

Christiane Northrup, *The Secret Pleasures of Menopause* (Hay House, 2008)
Henry Benson, *The Relaxation Response* (HarperTorch, 1975)
Louann Brizendine, *The Female Brain* (Broadway, 2006)

SELF-HELP

Jack Kornfield, *A Path with Heart: A Guide Through the Perils and Promises of Spiritual Life* (Bantam, 1993)

Marshall B. Rosenberg, *Nonviolent Communication: A Language of Life* (Gazelle, 2003)

Websites

To learn more about Audrey and her Restorative Yoga Training: https://restorativeyoga.org

To learn more about Judith Hanson Lasater: www.judithhansonlasater.com

To learn more about Lizzie Lasater: www.lizzielasater.com

To find a qualified Restorative Yoga teacher: www.restorativeyogateachers.com

Where to Find Yoga Props

These websites offer a variety of high-quality yoga props to support your practice.

Manduka: For bolsters, blankets, bricks, and straps, visit www.manduka.com and get 15 percent off using the coupon code RESTORATIVEREVOLUTION.

Yoga Matters: Explore www.yogamatters.com for bolsters, bricks, blocks, straps, and eye pillows.

Eye pillows: For lightweight soft eye pillows, visit http://eyepillows.it.

Hugger Mugger: Find bolsters and blankets at www.huggermugger.com.

Notes

Foreword

1 Judith Hanson Lasater, *Restore and Rebalance: Yoga for Deep Relaxation* (Shambhala, 2017), 37.

Preface

1 B. K. S. Iyengar, *Light on the Yoga Sutras of Patanjali* (HarperCollins, 1993).

Chapter 1: Where Does Restorative Yoga Come From?

1 Vimia Murthy and Kalyani Namjoshi, "Use of Props: An Interview with Guruji," Newsletter of the B. K. S. Iyengar Association of Australasia, March 1995, https://iyengaryogacentre.ca/wp-content/uploads/2019/07/7-newsletter_jul_aug_1995.pdf.

2 Donna Farhi, "Yoga's Culture of Abuse," RNZ, May 4, 2019, www.rnz.co.nz/national/programmes/saturday/audio/2018693565/donna-farhi-yoga-s-culture-of-abuse.

3 Donna Farhi, "Iyengar Abuse and Changing Yoga Pedagogy," J. Brown Yoga Talks, YouTube video, January 6, 2024, https://youtu.be/HTl7rlx38Yk?si=hlE6vjyG6E-ZVJ0v.

4 Jack Kornfield, *A Path with Heart: a Guide Through the Perils and Promises of Spiritual Life* (Bantam, 1993), 46.

5 Thomas H. Holmes and Richard H. Rahe, "The Social Readjustment Rating Scale," *Journal of Psychosomatic Research* 11:2 (August 1967), 213–18, https://doi.org/10.1016/0022-3999(67)90010-4.

6 Dominique Servant, Régis Logier, Y. Mouster, and Michel Goudemand, "La variabilité de la fréquence cardiaque. Intérêts en psychiatrie" [Heart rate variability. Applications in psychiatry], *L'Encéphale* 35:5 (October 2009), 423–28, https://doi.org/10.1016/j.encep.2008.06.016.

7 Navaz Habib, *Activez votre nerf vague: La nouvelle routine santé contre stress, inflammation, troubles digestifs, maladies auto-immunes* [Activate your vagus nerve: The new health routine against stress, inflammation, digestive issues, autoimmune diseases] (Thierry Souccar, 2020).

8 Edward Bullmore, *The Inflamed Mind: A Radical New Approach to Depression* (Picador, 2018).

9 Golam M. Khandaker, Rebecca M. Pearson, Stanley Zammit, Glyn Lewis, and Peter B. Jones, "Association of Serum Interleukin 6 and C-Reactive Protein in Childhood with Depression and Psychosis in Young Adult Life: A Population-Based Longitudinal Study," *JAMA Psychiatry* 71:10 (October 2014), 1121–28, https://doi.org/10.1001/jamapsychiatry.2014.1332.

10 Andrew H. Miller and Charles L. Raison, "The Role of Inflammation in Depression: From Evolutionary Imperative to Modern Treatment Target," *Nature Reviews: Immunology* 16:1 (January 2016), 22–34, https://doi.org/10.1038/nri.2015.5.

11 Lucile Capuron and Andrew H. Miller, "Immune System to Brain Signaling: Neuropsychopharmacological Implications," *Pharmacology & Therapeutics* 130:2 (February 2011), 226–38, https://doi.org/10.1016/j.pharmthera.2011.01.014.

12 Habib, *Activez votre nerf vague.*

13 Henry Benson, *The Relaxation Response* (HarperTorch, 1975).

14 Bruno Bonaz, "Propriétés anti-inflammatoires du nerf vague: implications thérapeutiques en gastroentérologie" [Anti-inflammatory properties of the vagus nerve: Therapeutic implications in gastroenterology], *Hepato-Gastro-entérologie Libérale* 3:3 (January 2015), 173–79, https://doi.org/10.4267/2042/56896.

15 Janice K. Kiecolt-Glaser, Lisa Christian, Heather Preston, Carrie R. Houts, William B. Malarkey, Charles F. Emery, and Ronald Glaser, "Stress, inflammation, and yoga practice," *Psychosomatic Medicine* 72:2 (February 2010), 113–21, https://doi.org/10.1097/PSY.0b013e3181cb9377.

16 Roger Cole, "Relaxation: Physiology and Practice," 2003, unpublished.

Chapter 2: What Is Restorative Yoga?

1 Roger Cole, "Relaxation: Physiology and Practice," 2003, unpublished.

2 Bo Forbes, *Yoga for Emotional Balance: Simple Practices to Help Relieve Anxiety and Depression* (Shambhala, 2011), 208, 232.

3 Beth E. Cohen, A. Ann Chang, Deborah Grady, and Alka M. Kanaya, "Restorative Yoga in Adults with Metabolic Syndrome: A Randomized, Controlled Pilot Trial," *Metabolic Syndrome and Related Disorders* 6:3 (September 2008), 223–29, https://doi.org/10.1089/met.2008.0016.

4 Mel Robin, *A Physiological Handbook for Teachers of Yogasana* (Fenestra, 2002), 218.

5 R. J. Cole, "Postural Baroreflex Stimuli May Affect EEG Arousal and Sleep in Humans," *Journal of Applied Physiology* 67:6 (December 1989), 2369–75, https://doi.org/10.1152/jappl.1989.67.6.2369.

6 Judith Hanson Lasater, *Yogabody: Anatomy, Kinesiology, and Asana* (Shambhala, 2009), 14.

7 Hatha Yoga Pradipika I:34.

Chapter 3: Cultivating Emotional Balance

1 Hatha Yoga Pradipika II:68.

2 Navaz Habib, *Activez votre nerf vague: La nouvelle routine santé contre stress, inflammation, troubles digestifs, maladies auto-immunes* [Activate your vagus nerve: The new health routine against stress, inflammation, digestive issues, autoimmune diseases] (Thierry Souccar, 2020), ch. 15.

3 Eddie Weitzberg and Jon O. N. Lundberg, "Humming Greatly Increases Nasal Nitric Oxide," *American Journal of Respiratory and Critical Care Medicine* 166: 2 (2002), 144–45, https://doi.org/10.1164/rccm.200202-138BC.

4 Judith Hanson Lasater and Ike K. Lasater, *What We Say Matters: Practicing Nonviolent Communication* (Shambhala, 2009).

5 Jillian Pransky, *Deep Listening: A Healing Practice to Calm Your Body, Clear Your Mind, and Open Your Heart* (Rodale, 2017).

6 Andrew H. Miller and Charles L. Raison, "The Role of Inflammation in Depression: From Evolutionary Imperative to Modern Treatment Target," *Nature Reviews: Immunology* 16:1 (2016), 22–34, https://doi.org/10.1038/nri.2015.5.

7 Nobuyuki Sudo, Yoichi Chida, Yuji Aiba, Junko Sonoda, Naomi Oyama, Xiao-Nian Yu, Chiharu Kubo, and Yasuhiro Koga, "Postnatal Microbial Colonization Programs the Hypothalamic–Pituitary–Adrenal System for Stress Response in Mice," *Journal of Physiology* 558:1 (2004) 263–75, https://doi.org/10.1113/jphysiol.2004.063388.

8 Mel Robin, *A Physiological Handbook for Teachers of Yogasana* (Fenestra, 2002), 205–6.

9 Bo Forbes, *Yoga for Emotional Balance: Simple Practices to Help Relieve Anxiety and Depression* (Shambhala, 2011), 19–20, 213.

10 Robin, *Physiological Handbook*, ch. 20.

11 Janette Zamudio Canales, Táki Athanássios Cordás, Juliana Teixeira Fiquer, André Furtado Cavalcante, and Ricardo Alberto Moreno, "Posture and Body Image in Individuals with Major Depressive Disorder: A Controlled Study," *Brazilian Journal of Psychiatry* 32:4 (2010), 375–80, https://doi.org/10.1590/s1516-44462010000400010.

12 Janice K. Kiecolt-Glaser, Lisa Christian, Heather Preston, Carrie R. Houts, William B. Malarkey, Charles F. Emery, and Ronald Glaser, "Stress, Inflammation, and Yoga Practice," *Psychosomatic Medicine* 72:2 (2010), 113–21, https://doi.org/10.1097/PSY.0b013e3181cb9377.

13 Mary Helen Immordino-Yang, Joanna A. Christodoulou, and Vanessa Singh, "Rest Is Not Idleness: Implications of the Brain's Default Mode for Human Development and Education," *Journal of the Association for Psychological Science* 7:4 (2012), 352–64, https://doi.org/10.1177/1745691612447308.

14 Michael Eggart, Andreas Lange, Martin J. Binser, Silvia Queri, and Bruno Müller-Oerlinghausen, "Major Depressive Disorder Is Associated with Impaired Interoceptive Accuracy: A Systematic Review," *Brain Sciences* 9:6 (2019), 131, https://doi.org/10.3390/brainsci9060131.

15 Vincenzo Monda, Ines Villano, Antonietta Messina, Anna Valenzano, Teresa Esposito, Fiorenzo Moscatelli, Andrea Viggiano, et al., "Exercise Modifies the Gut Microbiota with Positive Health Effects," *Oxidative Medicine and Cellular Longevity* 2017:3831972, https://doi.org/10.1155/2017/3831972; Valeriy A. Poroyko, Alba Carreras, Abdelnaby Khalyfa, Ahamed A. Khalyfa, Vanessa Leone, Eduard Peris, Isaac Almendros, et al., "Chronic Sleep Disruption Alters Gut Microbiota, Induces Systemic and Adipose Tissue Inflammation and Insulin Resistance in Mice," *Scientific Reports* 2016:35405 (2016). https://doi.org/10.1038/srep35405.

16 Kristin Neff, *Self-Compassion: The Proven Power of Being Kind to Yourself* (HarperCollins, 2011).

Chapter 4: Nurturing Well-Being Through Hormonal Shifts

1 Louann Brizendine, *The Female Brain* (Broadway, 2006).

2 Claudia Welch, *Balance Your Hormones, Balance Your Life: Achieving Optimal Health and Wellness through Ayurveda, Chinese Medicine, and Western Science* (Da Capo, 2011), 18.

3 Beth E. Cohen, Alka M. Kanaya, Judith L. Macer, Hui Shen, A. Ann Chang, and Deborah Grady, "Feasibility and Acceptability of Restorative Yoga for Treatment of Hot Flushes: A Pilot Trial," *Maturitas* 56:2 (2007), 198–204, https://doi.org/10.1016/j.maturitas.2006.08.003.

4 Judith Hanson Lasater, *Relax and Renew: Restful Yoga for Stressful Times* (Rodmell, 1995; repr. Shambhala, 2016).

5 Jillian Pransky, *Deep Listening: A Healing Practice to Calm Your Body, Clear Your Mind, and Open Your Heart* (Rodale, 2017), 167–68.

6 Courtney Denning-Johnson Lynch, Rajeshwari Sundaram, José M. Maisog, A. M. Sweeney, and Germaine M. Buck Louis, "Preconception Stress Increases the Risk of Infertility: Results from a Couple-Based Prospective Cohort Study—the LIFE Study," *Human Reproduction* 29:5 (March 2014), https://doi.org/10.1093/humrep/deu032.

7 Geeta S. Iyengar, *Yoga: A Gem for Women* (1983; 3rd rev. ed. New Delhi: Allied, 2019), 237.

8 Judith Hanson Lasater, *Yoga Myths: What You Need to Learn and Unlearn for a Safe and Healthy Yoga Practice* (Shambhala, 2020), 175.

9 Ellen B. Gold, Sybil L. Crawford, Nancy E. Avis, Carolyn J. Crandall, Karen A. Matthews, L. Elaine Waetjen, Jennifer S. Lee, et al., "Factors Related to Age at Natural Menopause: Longitudinal Analyses From SWAN," *American Journal of Epidemiology* 178:1 (2013), 70–83, https://doi.org/10.1093/aje/kws421.

10 Claudia Welch, *Balance Your Hormones, Balance Your Life: Achieving Optimal Health and Wellness through Ayurveda, Chinese Medicine, and Western Science* (Da Capo, 2011), 32.

11 Nancy E. Avis, Sybil L. Crawford, Gail Greendale, Joyce T. Bromberger, Susan A. Everson-Rose, Ellen B. Gold, Rachel Hess, et al., "Duration of Menopausal Vasomotor Symptoms over the Menopause Transition," *JAMA Internal Medicine* 175:4 (2015), 531–39, https://doi.org/10.1001/jamainternmed.2014.8063.

12 Beth E. Cohen et al., "Restorative Yoga for Treatment of Hot Flushes."

About the Author

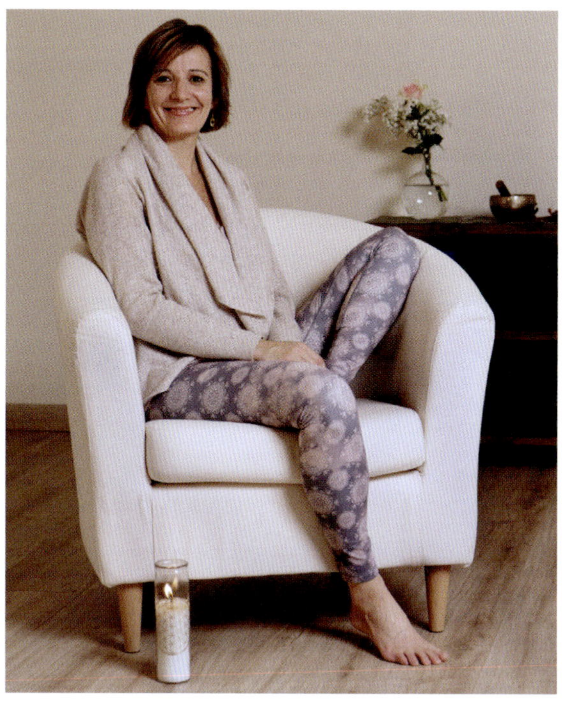

Originally from France and living amidst the picturesque Monferrato Hills of Italy, **Audrey Favreau** is a passionate Restorative Yoga teacher trainer and certified professional coach. Her journey to becoming a leader in the field of Restorative Yoga is deeply rooted in her own transformative experiences.

Audrey holds a master's degree in the Science of Management from Audencia Nantes and a professional certification in private and business coaching from Coach & Team. She spent eleven years working as a manager for a leading French bank, enduring the weight of chronic stress. Discovering Restorative Yoga became a turning point in her life, offering profound healing and inspiring her to share this life-changing practice with others.

As a certified E-RYT 200 yoga teacher through Yoga Alliance, a YACEP (Yoga Alliance Continuing Education Provider), and a Relax and Renew Advanced Trainer, Audrey brings a wealth of knowledge and expertise to her teachings.

Since 2015 she has trained and inspired hundreds of students, empowering them to embrace the art of relaxation and integrate Restorative Yoga into their lives.

In addition to teaching, Audrey is a regular contributor to Italian magazine *Vivere lo Yoga*, where she shares her insights and expertise on Restorative Yoga. Audrey's vision is simple yet powerful: a world where everyone learns to slow down, embrace rest, and experience the profound physical and emotional benefits of Restorative Yoga. Her work continues to inspire people to prioritize self-care and transform their lives through the art of relaxation.

About North Atlantic Books

North Atlantic Books (NAB) is an independent, nonprofit publisher committed to a bold exploration of the relationships between mind, body, spirit, and nature. Founded in 1974, NAB aims to nurture a holistic view of the arts, sciences, humanities, and healing. To make a donation or to learn more about our books, authors, events, and newsletter, please visit www.northatlanticbooks.com.